ART FOR YOUR SANITY

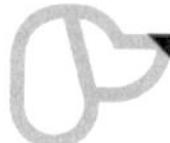

SH&H Publishing

Contact information for SH&H Publishing LLC – susan@susan-hensley.com

Library of Congress Control Number: 2024907276

ISBN: 979-8-218-38898-0 (paperback)
ISBN: 979-8-218-38899-7 (ebook)

Ordering Information:
Special discounts are available on quantity purchases by corporations, associations, and others. For details, contact susan@susan-hensley.com

Publisher's Cataloging-in-Publication Data
Names: Hensley, Susan, 1964- .
Title: Art for your sanity : how art journaling can help you manage chaos and unleash joy / Susan Hensley.
Description: Austin, TX : SH&H Publications, 2024. | Includes index. | Includes color photos. | Summary: Presents art journaling as a journey of self-discovery and renewal, and a tool for managing the chaos of change.
Identifiers: LCCN X | ISBN 9798218388980 (pbk.) | ISBN 9798218388997 (ebook)
Subjects: LCSH: Art therapy. | Creation (Literary, artistic, etc.). | Diaries – Authorship – Technique. | Stress management. | BISAC: SELF-HELP / Creativity. | SELF-HELP / Journaling. | ART / Techniques / General.
Classification: LCC RC489.A7 H46 2024 | DDC 745.593 H--dc23
LC record available at https://lccn.loc.gov/X

ART FOR YOUR SANITY

How Art Journaling Can Help You Manage Chaos and Unleash Joy

SUSAN HENSLEY

DEDICATION

This book is dedicated to those who have the courage to live a life that is wild, free, and filled with joy.

CONTENTS

DEAR READER

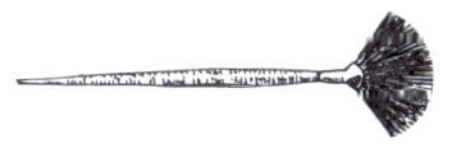

IT MIGHT SOUND LIKE HYPERBOLE WHEN I SAY THAT MY ART JOURNAL IS MY GPS, best friend, sounding board, and wisest confidant. But that declaration is no exaggeration. My art journal has grown to be all those things and more. I can safely say that art journaling got me through the COVID-19 pandemic and all the fear and anxiety I felt during that time. It helped me access the wisdom within myself to know when it was time to retire and move on from my role at a company I had loved for more than two decades. And when this transition brought on anxiety, art journaling empowered me to jump into retirement with no real plan.

When I started art journaling, I had no idea it would be such a huge source of self-discovery. Art journaling gives my inner "knowing" a voice that can speak directly to me. Each new page gives form to that place of wisdom and stillness, allowing my spirit to come through and guide me—a truly profound impact. But perhaps what surprised me the most was how much fun I had on each page. I would never have thought that two such distinct words—profound and fun—could coexist harmoniously and impactfully in a single activity until I adopted art journaling.

In addition to fun, when it felt like I was jumping off a metaphorical cliff in making a major life transition, art journaling kept me sane and hopeful. It helped create clarity during the discomfort of change and transition. My art journal became the only place where my mind went to play, and that play taught me to trust my longings. It showed me that intriguing and wonderful insights can emerge from one simple art page, which more often than not looks like a completely misshapen mess of color and shapes.

Art journaling helps me "lighten up," to get inside my "right brain" and move out of my overthinking, overanxious left brain, even if only for just a few minutes.

Believe me, I never set out to publish a book on art journaling or a compilation of personal essays on how art journaling has helped me through a major transition. Rather, I simply feel compelled to follow what the art journal is telling me as it applies to my daily life. Still, I almost can't *not* publish this book. As a recovering perfectionist and people-pleaser, the insights and fun I experienced through art journaling during a major life transition are far too great to not publish and share.

So here it goes. I hope this book helps you find fun and explore new insights through your art journal. Most of all, I hope you'll rediscover your inner child artist—you know, the one who creates for the sheer joy of creation, who has not yet met their inner critic, the one who trusts that what may look like a mess on a page is actually a masterpiece of self-discovery.

I suggest having a notebook handy as you read this book to capture thoughts, feelings, and situations you may want to express in your art journal. At the end of each section, I've included a few prompts to help you get started. Remember there are no rights or wrongs in this process. You are creating your own private place for discovery and play.

Have fun!

Susan Hensley

INTRODUCTION

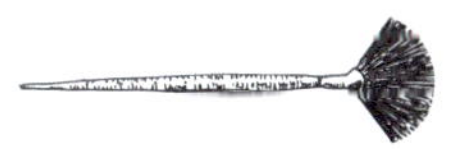

AS ADULTS, WE HAVE A POWER LONG LOST IN THE DEMANDS OF THE hustle and bustle of everyday life. That power stems from the simplicity and authenticity of a child's perspective, untainted by societal conditioning. Childhood wisdom is the true name of such power.

Curiosity and playfulness reign supreme in our early years, and imagination knows no bounds. Children view the world with wonder, finding joy in the simplest of things, and approaching challenges with resilience. Their unfettered honesty and intuitive understanding of emotions allow them to navigate complex situations with a clarity often lost with age. The power of childhood wisdom lies in its ability to remind us of the fundamental truths: to embrace curiosity, find joy in the mundane, approach life with resilience, and value genuine connections above all. Harnessing that wisdom can rekindle creativity, resilience, and a sense of wonder often buried beneath the layers of adulthood complexities.

Life transitions can bring us to our knees with anxious thoughts, worries, and endless internal debates about what we should or could be doing. Art journaling—a visual diary of your emotions, thoughts, dreams, and fears fueled by your inner artist—can prove a powerful tool during challenging stages of our lives when we need a way to step back from the angst and tap into that childhood wisdom. It provides a fun, supportive place to move from endless worry and rumination to a place of joyful anticipation and childlike curiosity. Each element of art journaling moves us into our right brain, where there is space to explore and problem-solve without the linear constraints of the left brain. It also silences our inner critic, opening the door to a playful abode bountiful with the insight needed to guide us through any life transition.

DISCLAIMER

The content provided herein is intended for informational purposes only and represents my own journey through art journaling. It is not intended to substitute for professional advice, diagnosis, or treatment. While my words may touch upon aspects related to psychology or wellness, it is crucial to note that this content should not be considered as art therapy or a replacement for professional therapy or counseling services. Always seek the advice of qualified professionals regarding any mental health or therapeutic needs.

Part One

ART JOURNALING

What is art journaling? Can anyone do it?
What if I'm not creative or artistic? What tools do I need?

ONE

A HOBBY WITH NO STRINGS ATTACHED

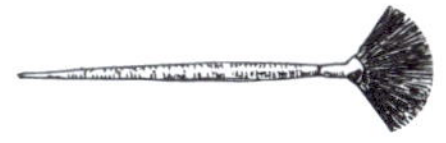

ART JOURNALING ARRIVED IN MY LIFE DURING A TIME WHEN I REALLY needed a hobby. And not just any hobby, something stress-free, convenient, creative, and enriching.

I've never felt I had hobbies, at least not in the way I think of other people as having hobbies, such as sports, music, painting, etc. Sure, I had passions and interests, but they weren't what I thought of as a true hobby. I consulted my trusty friend, Google, for the definition of "hobby" and saw that I probably did have hobbies—reading, travel, exercise. However, none of those hobbies really tapped into my creative side, my expressive side. I sort of wondered what was wrong with me. I was also worried as I contemplated the endless hours of available free time that were looming for me in my mid-50s and beyond as my retirement drew closer.

At the time, I had such huge responsibility and was under loads of pressure at work. The world was in the throes of the pandemic. I was overwhelmed with stress because I was working in human resources. So, as you can imagine, I was working huge, huge amounts at that time. Any person in HR was pulling their hair out during the pandemic. It was challenging work, to put it mildly, and especially at the company where I was working because half of the workforce—the manufacturing crew—had to be in-office and the other half of the staff didn't. That situation was an unbelievable challenge in a company with over 7,000 employees. The constantly changing policies and regulations were a complete nightmare, not to mention that there was a deadly rogue virus on the loose.

So, there I was, working a stressful HR position (remotely for the first time) during one of the worst pandemics in modern history. I was quarantined away from my friends, family, and coworkers. I was at my wit's end. The hobbies I relied on were no longer sufficient to stem my unease. I couldn't travel, and I couldn't go to yoga or Pilates. And although I love reading, there's really only so much reading one can do, right? Given that I was about to retire, my anxiety over what I was going to do in the next stage of my life added to the overwhelming state of being homebound.

I needed to *do* something—something fun and colorful. Shortly before the pandemic, a friend of mine took up painting after she broke her ankle and was laid up for weeks. She learned to practice her art technics in a journal format and shared the process in the form of mini-workshops. There, she and many other artists focused on their specific craft and enhancing their skill. When I went to one of her weekend introductions to art journaling, though, I was more intrigued by how art journaling could help me in life transitions. I immediately felt art journaling wouldn't be about my developing as an artist, but rather helping me process emotions and navigate the chaos that comes with life transitions. I was tired of drab and dreary, and I wasn't doing well having been so isolated during the quarantine period. The whimsical, childlike play that I experienced in the workshop called to me.

Art journaling began to fill my need to counteract the current pressures all around me. I remembered times past in my ordinary days when I had frequently started doodling in spare moments. Now, I saw doodling as a way to return to a tactic that would relieve the distress of anxiety and calm my mind.

Then, during longer breaks in my workday, I took out the colored pencils from my younger years and began drawing shapes and images in a notebook I had handy. I immediately noticed the calm surrounding me.

Once I started art journaling regularly, color returned to those seemingly endless days. I quickly realized another perk of art journaling; it was just for me. In my world of constant helping, working, and just plain giving of myself to the point of depletion, this diversion was huge.

I also appreciated that art journaling went beyond interest and distraction. It sparked joy and gave me a feeling of clean energy, free from the pressure of my other hobbies. With them, the "shoulds" get overwhelming: I should read this type of book, I should aim for hobbies that are social, or I should only pick intellectual hobbies, etc. Or even worse, we tell ourselves "I should be better at this." But art journaling freed me from all of those "shoulds." I could say, "No, I'm going to stay right at my four-year-old self, thank you very much."

We all turn to hobbies for different reasons. But I think that as adults, we often pick hobbies that allow us to numb ourselves from the stress of the world around us. And numbing isn't always a good thing. Hobbies like art journaling, which is purely for play, are ideal. And art journaling has the extra bonus of personal development—self-discovery, understanding our emotions, and helping us learn more about ourselves.

TWO

HOW TO GET STARTED WITH ART JOURNALING

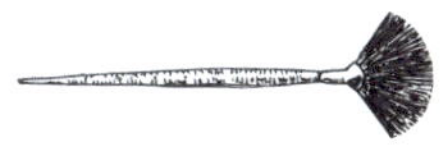

AS I SAID EARLIER, I TRAVELED AS A HOBBY, AND I LOVE TO TRAVEL. I'D actually consider it my favorite hobby. As enriching as it is, it's not exactly something I can just pull out of a drawer, do for five minutes, and then put away when I'm done. Art journaling is pure relaxation of mind, and who doesn't need that? It allows me to doodle on impulse for five minutes and still feel as if I traveled to Rome. Well, okay, maybe not Rome exactly, but I think you get my point.

Best yet, art journaling is easy to start and inexpensive. You don't need fancy equipment—just a couple of magazines, an Elmers glue stick (the big fat kind), a notebook, some basic watercolors (the pan type we used as kids), some gel pens, and colored pencils or crayons. In fact, I completely skipped Amazon and art supply stores, which are stocked with "real" art stuff. Instead, I headed straight to the kids' school-supply section at Target. I just whisked through, grabbing random kid art supplies and then, presto! I was officially ready to start my art journaling.

I encourage you to join the colorful world of art journaling! Just remember: This is your art journal, so make it your own! For me, having the variety of childhood art tools is what really makes art journaling fun and playful, but may I suggest the following few tips when choosing items that call to you.

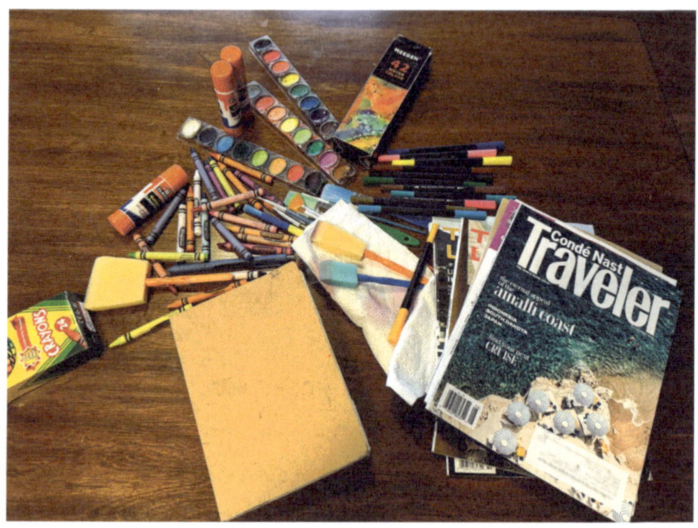

My art journaling supplies. These are similar to what I used when I was a child. Keeping my supplies simple helps me stay playful and creative and keeps my inner perfectionist on the sidelines.

NOTEBOOK

The first must-have item is a notebook. You can make your own with a simple three-ring binder and some paper, you can use an old blank book, planner, etc. You'll want the pages to be blank—lined pages might limit your creative process.

If you're going to purchase a notebook, I recommend either a notebook with spiral binding or a standard notebook that lays flat. I choose not to use a spiral because sometimes I span across two pages, so I like bound books, but again, your preference wins here.

I also prefer a notebook that's sized such that it fits easily in a purse or backpack, so I use 5.7x8. It keeps it handy.

Paper thickness is important, too. You'll want a notebook with paper that's thick enough to manage glue, watercolor, and heavier paints. If you plan on just sketching and doodling, then thickness doesn't matter.

PAINTS

I use watercolor paints. They're messy until they dry, but that's the best part about them. They roll everywhere, which provides me with the thrill of watching how they move because the color changes and spreads as it dries. Plus, watercolors are the easiest paints to collage over and around.

My best friend gave me really beautiful watercolors, which have rich pigment, but I find my favorite watercolors really are Crayola's. They're easy and fast, which is important in art journaling because this hobby is also meant to be spontaneous for moments when you need a refreshing break.

GLUE

Glue sticks make things feel really playful. I choose to use the really wide Elmer's glue sticks because they have more surface area.

PENCILS, PENS, AND CRAYONS

Gel pens are easy to keep in my purse and to store in various places around the house, so these are my go to. Their colors are beautiful, and they're easy to use. I also use crayons, just the simple Crayola-type we used when we were kids. Some people use paint pens, fine liner pens, and colored pencils, all of which are great options, too. Go with your gut.

COLLAGE MATERIALS

Collage is incredibly fun and easy, and my go-to supply for it is old magazines. But you could use vintage ephemera, tissue paper (which you can see through and makes a cool effect), construction paper, or scrapbooking papers (metallic, colorful, patterned, etc.). Try saving pretty gift wrapping and consider greeting cards, and not just the front but what people have written to you inside the cards as well. You can get super creative here.

THREE

WHAT TO DO WHEN YOU DON'T KNOW WHERE TO START

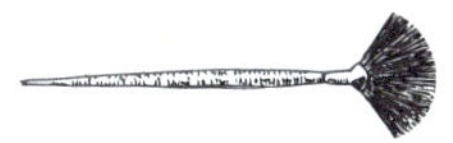

BEGINNING IS THE HARDEST PART OF ANY NEW ACTIVITY OR HOBBY. SO, I'LL give a few pointers here, too. I recommend starting with collage.

Cut out images or phrases that speak to you. Then try arranging them on the page in a way that makes you feel good. Decorate those pages with paint, markers, paper, or any of your other supplies. During the entire process, continuously check in with yourself. How do you feel? Is anything coming up for you? What colors, shapes, or magazine pictures are calling to you? Again, go with your gut. Start small and see where it takes you.

Another way to start is to look back and recall what medium of art you loved as a kid (water colors, crayons, colored pens/pencils, glue) and start there. Then think of images or shapes you liked to draw as a kid (flowers, trees, people, houses, cats, dogs, etc.). I used to draw hearts and smiley faces and still enjoy drawing them today. Did you or do you have a go-to doodle?

Initially, and until the process gets more comfortable, quickly jump into the page with whatever medium (stickers, crayons, paints, pens, collaging) feels good. Don't be afraid to work with a couple of pages at a time. I am surprised at what I find when I work across several pages using different colors that seem right in the moment. Keep in mind that the end creation is not the goal—it's the process that matters.

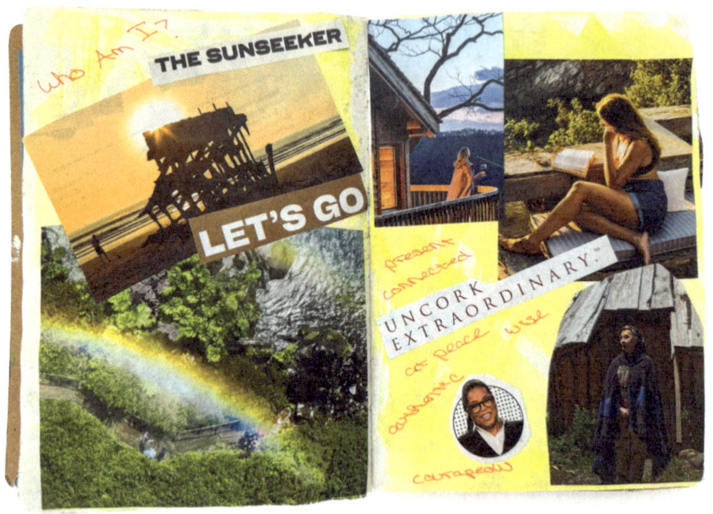

A collage I made after I announced my retirement. The question "Who am I?" filled pages and pages in my journal in the following months. I chose this color because although I felt uncertain, I wanted to feel the sunny optimism of yellow.

Still feel stuck? That's okay! Here are a few more tips to get the playfulness flowing:

- Gather some magazines and tear out any picture that is interesting to you. Remember, this is not a vision board, it's just pictures you like. I highly suggest travel magazines, given the beauty of the photography.
- Consider painting with your fingers, swirling paint. Get

messy and see if that increases your sense of play.

- If you're upset or uncertain how you feel, choose colors that represent your mood and start playing with them. See if words come to mind that describe the colors or what shapes go with the colors.
- Take a walk outside. Do you see a flower, or a leaf, or an expanse of colors that intrigue you or that you find particularly pleasing? Then, use watercolors, particularly because they are messy and spread quickly, and work with those colors, letting them blend into one another.
- Cut out words from magazines that speak to you. Sort through them and use them as a personal one-word prompt for art journaling. They sell decks of cards on the internet if you want, but it could be fun for you to cut out your own words and see what they inspire.
- Use a positive affirmation about yourself and use colors, pictures, or stickers to journal what that affirmation feels like to you. For example, if I feel grateful, I might like gathering pictures of presents. Others might feel like drawing the sun or stars. Feeling brave? I might choose pictures of someone who is strong. Feeling adventurous? I might look for pictures of a waterfall or a mountain, or draw them myself. You get the idea.
- What does the time of day or time of year look like or feel like to you? Is there an upcoming holiday or season that inspires you? Choose images that represent such feelings.
- Another good prompt is to think of favorite songs. How would you represent the feeling from the music through color or pictures?
- How do you feel when you think of loved ones or of people

open
hearts
prepare to be
delighted

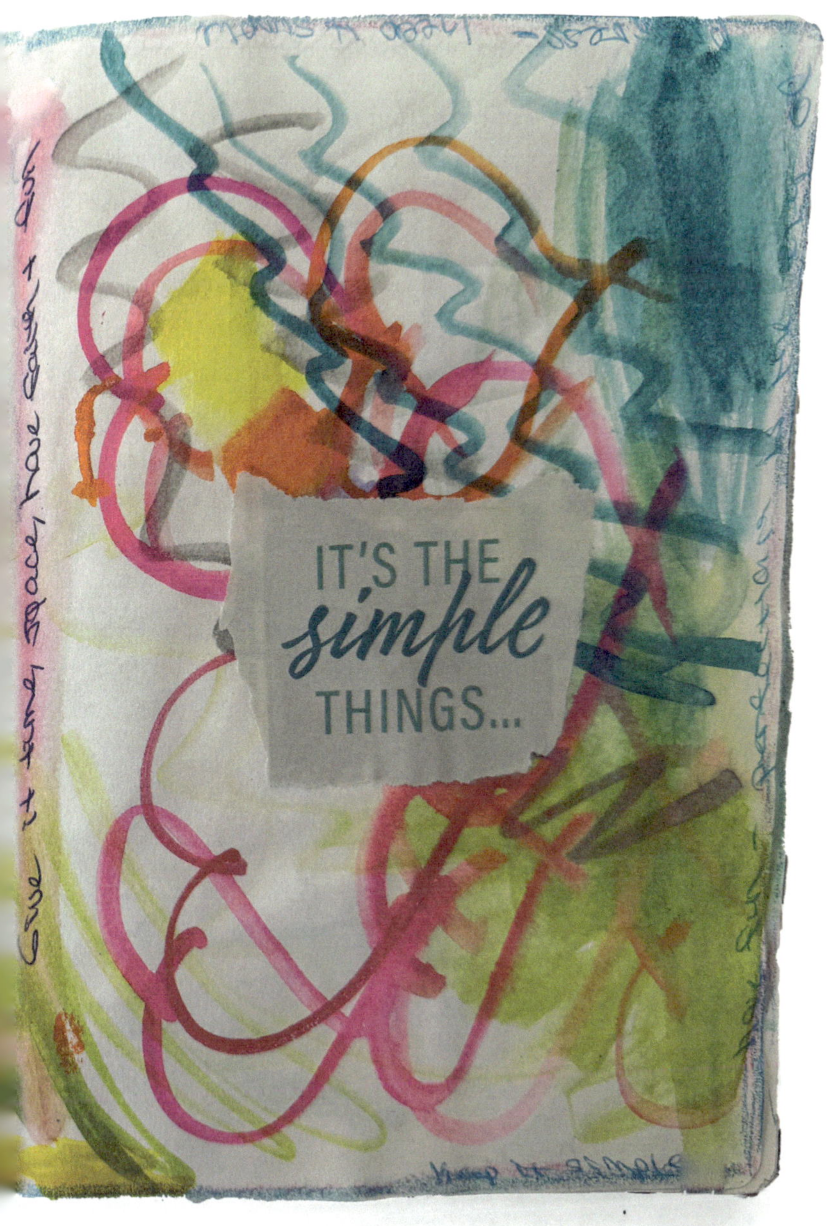

A journal entry while sitting in a coffee shop. This one always makes me smile.

with whom you have a difficult relationship? Use colors, materials, and art media to journal the effect of such relationships.

The most important point is that your art journal is just for you. It is as private as your written diary/journal. Don't overthink what you are drawing/creating. It should feel either fun and playful or like a release when it comes to dealing with difficult emotions.

Try art journaling at different times of day, in different moods for at least a month—my first attempts were filled with judgment. It wasn't until I started thinking of it as my personal playpen that I really started to have fun.

Just remember to keep it playful. Always playful. There are some days when I open a blank page, and the next thing I know, I am drawing different colored hearts, and I am happy. I am playing. I have no agenda, goal, or real thought. I am simply creating images that make me happy—in many cases hearts and smiley faces. I feel free and four years old again, safe and secure in the world.

My biggest piece of advice is to make a complete mess!

Part Two

A PLACE FOR PLAY AND FUN

Art journaling is a fun place to play with color and images that make you feel good.

FOUR

PLAY? WHAT'S THAT?

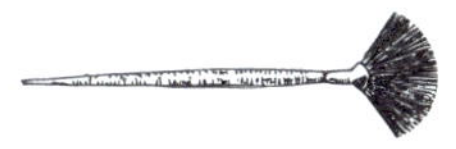

IN THEIR BOOK *DESIGNING YOUR LIFE: HOW TO BUILD A WELL-LIVED, Joyful Life*, Stanford University professors Bill Burnett and Dave Evans show us how to break free from the 9–5 shackles of our job to find our true calling, the one that fills you with passion, purpose, and fulfillment. The book includes an interesting exercise called the Love-Play-Work-Health Dashboard, a life-design exercise intended to help their readers get an accurate reading of where they're at in life right now in regard to the "four main pillars" of life: health, work, play, and love.

When partaking in this exercise, most people discover that they have adequate (or close to adequate, anyway) balance in the health, work, and love pillars of their lives. However, many adults are seriously deficient in the play pillar. Burnett and Evans define play as things we do just for fun; the things you do just because they make you happy, not for merit or improvement.

We all know that play provides a key role in child development, and kids naturally know how to play. As adults, though, we tend to view play as a foreign construct or at least a long-forgotten one. But pure play—doing something enjoyable solely for the enjoyment of it—is so important to our health and well-being. Researchers have found that play makes us more creative, sharpens our sense of humor, and help us better cope with stress. Art journaling is an ideal way to play. Its delightfully unstructured nature allows us to rediscover play without judgment from self or others.

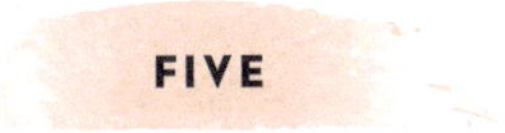

FIVE

ART JOURNALING AS A PLACE FOR PLAY

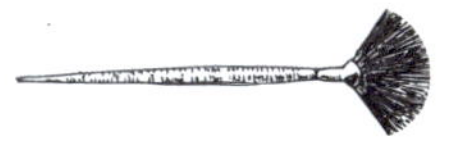

"You can discover more about a person in an hour of play than in a year of conversation."

—PROVERB

ART JOURNALING IS AN IDEAL PLAYGROUND FOR AN ADULT, ALLOWING you to play with colors, textures, and ideas in a relaxed, unstructured way. Playing in my art journal is handy and convenient, giving it a low "barrier to entry," so to speak. I can keep my art journal in my bag or purse and pull it out any time I need to spend a few minutes getting lost in my four-year-old self.

It encourages playful exploration of thoughts, ideas, and feelings without strict rules or boundaries. Images, colors, and words allow us to freely and playfully tap into our childlike selves to express emotions, thoughts, and ideas in a powerful way. We can reflect on our experiences, growth, and aspirations through artful expression and with childlike wonder. It helps us to access the joy and curiosity of the inner child, embracing spontaneity and fun.

Again, there's no right or wrong in art journaling; it's about the process, not the outcome. It's playtime for the soul, letting you unwind, explore, and discover without the pressure of perfection.

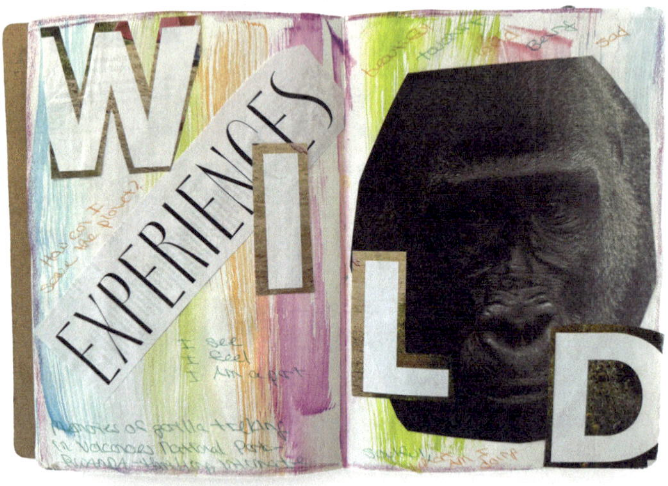

This entry captured the full range of emotions for me—memories of a favorite trip, my love of animals, my love of nature, and my fears about climate change. I was feeling it all.

SIX

THE CREATIVITY MYTH

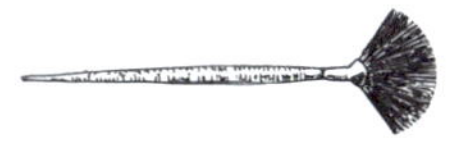

I FIND THE BIGGEST HURDLE THAT PEOPLE HAVE TO REDISCOVERING PLAY in art journaling is this statement: "I'm just not a creative person."

If that's you, you're not alone. I've heard that every three out of four people think they're not creative. General estimates and studies suggest that a significant portion of the population, roughly around 70% to 75%, have doubts about their creative abilities or consider themselves not particularly creative.

In my opinion, the definition of creativity is often too narrow. People who associate creativity only with the outcome—that in order to be "creative" you have to create an end product that is "original"—leave the process out of the equation. Such a belief places the emphasis on the outcome as opposed to the process. Dr. Ignacio L. Götz, author and researcher, argues that creativity is the act of creating without thinking about the end product, saying that one can be creative without necessarily being original.

SEVEN

HOW TO FIRE UP YOUR PLAYFUL NATURE

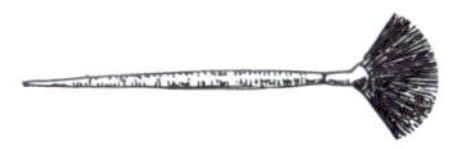

THE KEY TO BEING PLAYFUL IN ART JOURNALING IS TO REMOVE THE outcome from the equation and focus on the process…to create simply for the enjoyment of creating. When you follow that practice, you can drop the fear baggage—fear of judgment, criticism, and failure. The piece that you create is for your private enjoyment, not for others' approval.

Focusing on the process in art journaling also removes the pressure to meet societal standards of art and creativity. As kids, we learn early on whether or not we are "creatives" or "artists." Susan Magsamen and Ivy Ross say it well in their book *Your Brain on Art*: "Somewhere around third grade you may have received the message from a teacher, or other adult in your life, that you couldn't be an artist if you didn't have talent. And you also figured out that creativity was not as important as getting the answers correct on the endless bubble tests in school."

I'll tell you something important: Art journaling has zero to do with being "creative" or "artistic" and everything to do with self-dis-

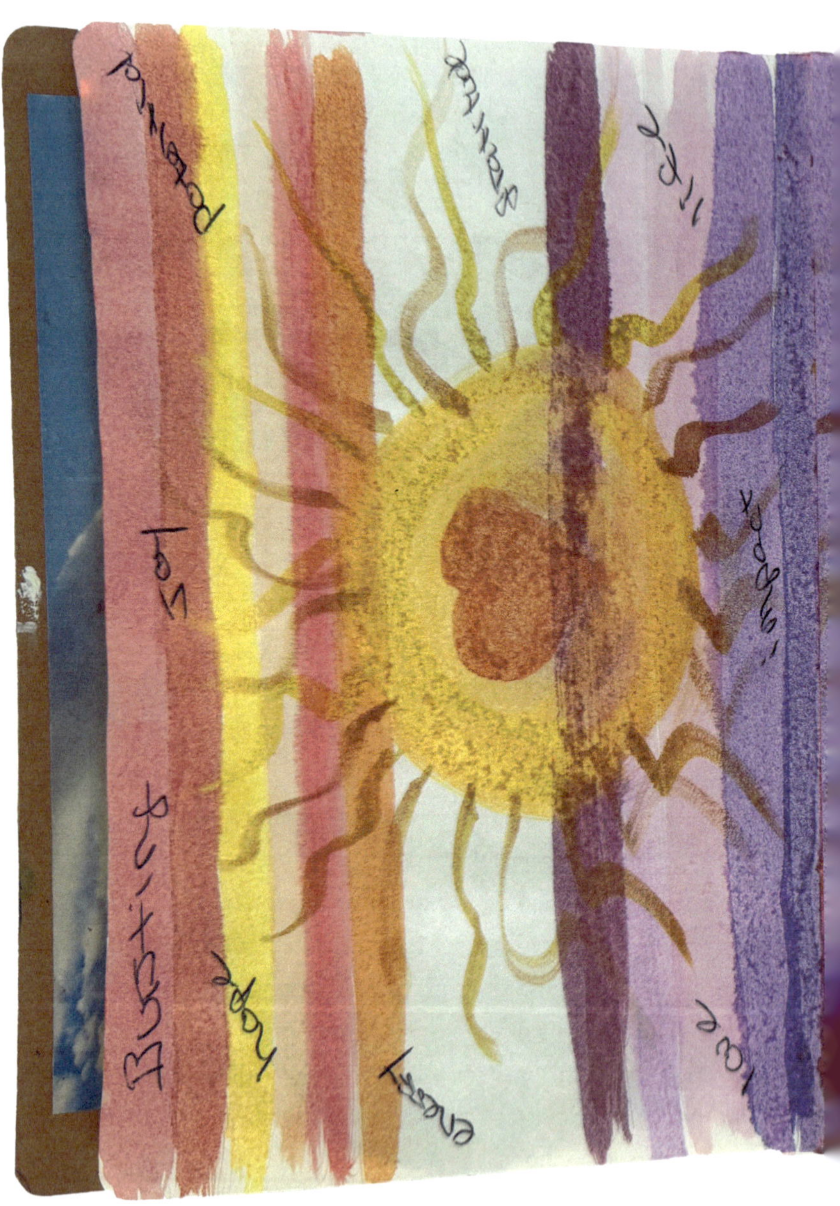
potential
gratitude
life
Bursting
joy
support
hope
energy
love

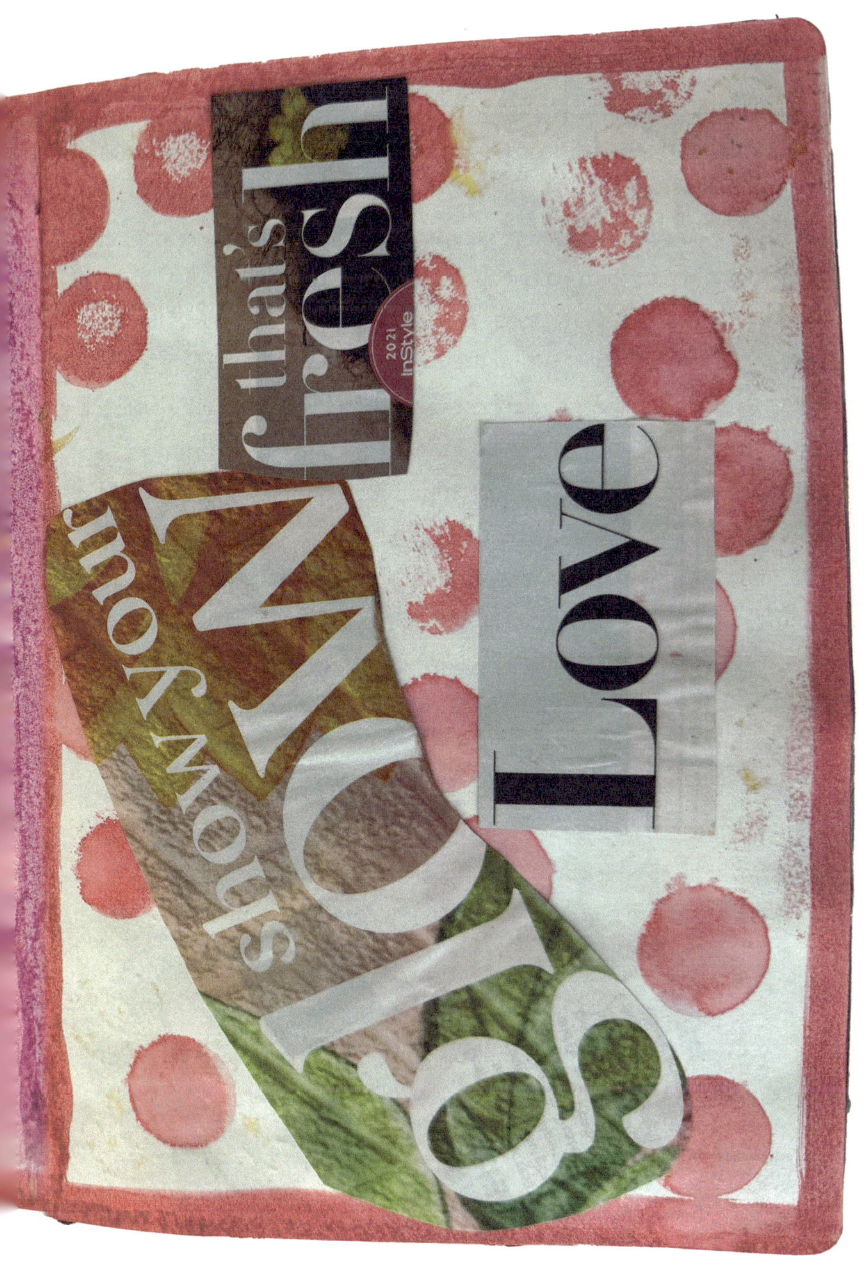

Play time. This page continues to boost my spirits whenever I see it.

covery, self-soothing, and just plain old fun.

Your Brain on Art also contains a very pertinent quote by Nicholas Wilton, artist and founder of Art2Life: "Art-making is, really, about feeling more alive in your life. The creative path is an unfolding process of becoming ourselves, and it's a wonderful journey we get to take." I couldn't agree more with that statement. Every page in my art journal is a path to self-discovery.

The authors go on to say, "The biggest deterrent to embracing our innate artistic selves is the inner critic that shuts down our creativity. It's our human need to know what we're doing, where we're going, and our desire to be good at it." According to Wilton, overcoming those tendencies requires "reframing art-making as a process of becoming yourself, and the things that you're making along the way are just the artifacts of that process."

My advice is to abandon your adult brain for a spell and take a breather from your usual industrious self by drawing or coloring. You'll fire up your playful nature, and I guarantee you'll see the benefits!

Let's take a moment and think about what types of drawings you created as a child. What types of things did you enjoy drawing? Did you draw animals? How about nature, such as flowers or trees? Did you draw people or fantastical creatures?

Pull out your notebook and whatever supplies you have nearby, such as colored pens, crayons, or even a pencil, and start drawing. Feel free to set a timer for 10 minutes and have fun. There's no judgment. Tap into that natural place of childlike play!

Part Three

A TOOL FOR LIFE TRANSITIONS

Art journaling is a great source of self-knowledge and can provide subconscious guidance about how to move forward during periods of life transitions.

EIGHT

FINDING PEACE WITH UNCERTAINTY

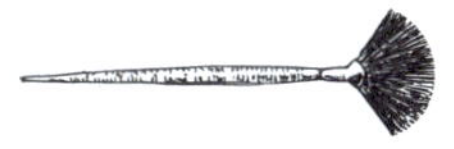

MEYER HOWARD ABRAMS ONCE SAID, "LIFE IS A JOURNEY UP A SPIRAL staircase." But when I'm facing a life transition, I wish I had a GPS telling me exactly where to go and when to turn, as well as when I would arrive. There is something so reassuring about that voice from a guidance system telling us where to turn, which lane to be in, and even warning about hazards in the area. If only transitioning through stages of life could be as straightforward, right?

With a GPS you just enter where you want to be at the end, and it takes you there. Of course, with a GPS you need to know where you are headed; life transitions are not always that clear. You go forward during a transition a step at a time, unsure with many of those steps if you are headed in the right direction or are going in circles. And of course, there is fear of getting stuck and going nowhere. The best part of a GPS, though, is it always allows us to ask for a new route or, heck, just enter a new destination.

Not so with life. Our life journeys are not so easily guided, and sometimes our choices are restricted. Often, we must navigate to

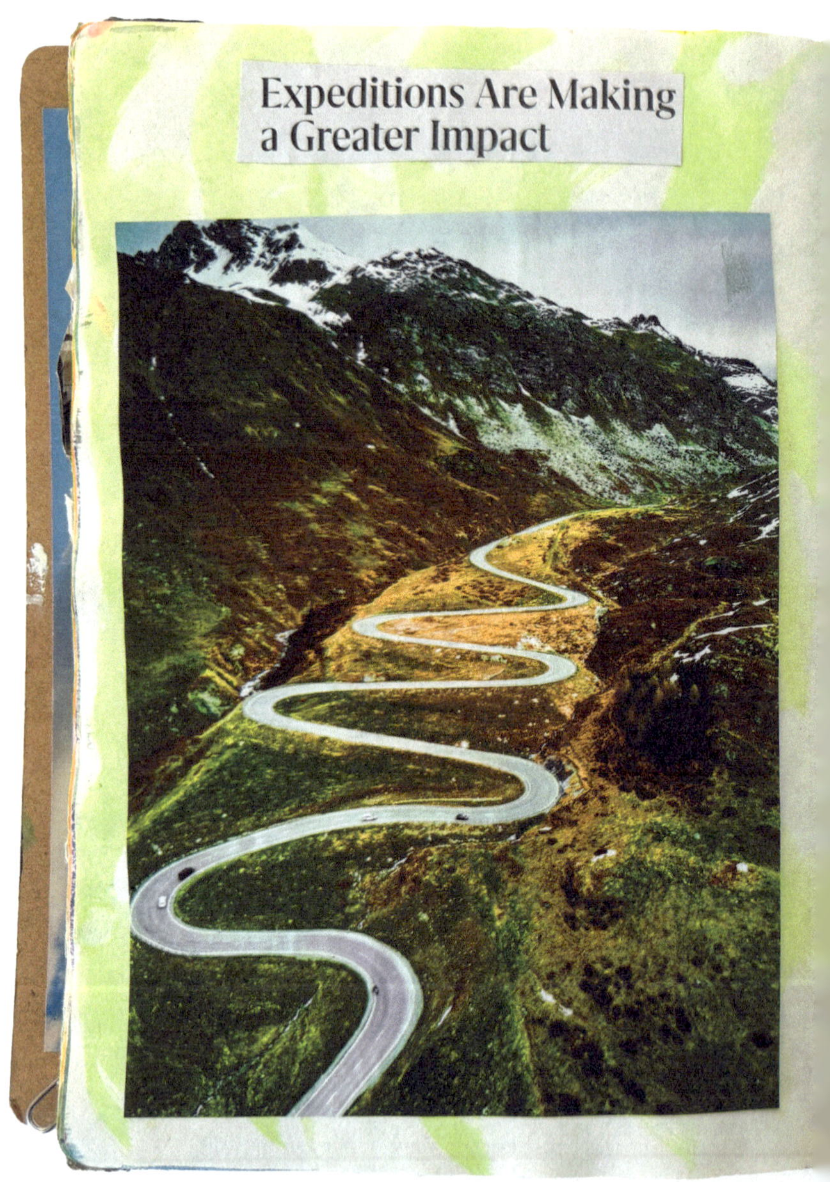
Expeditions Are Making
a Greater Impact

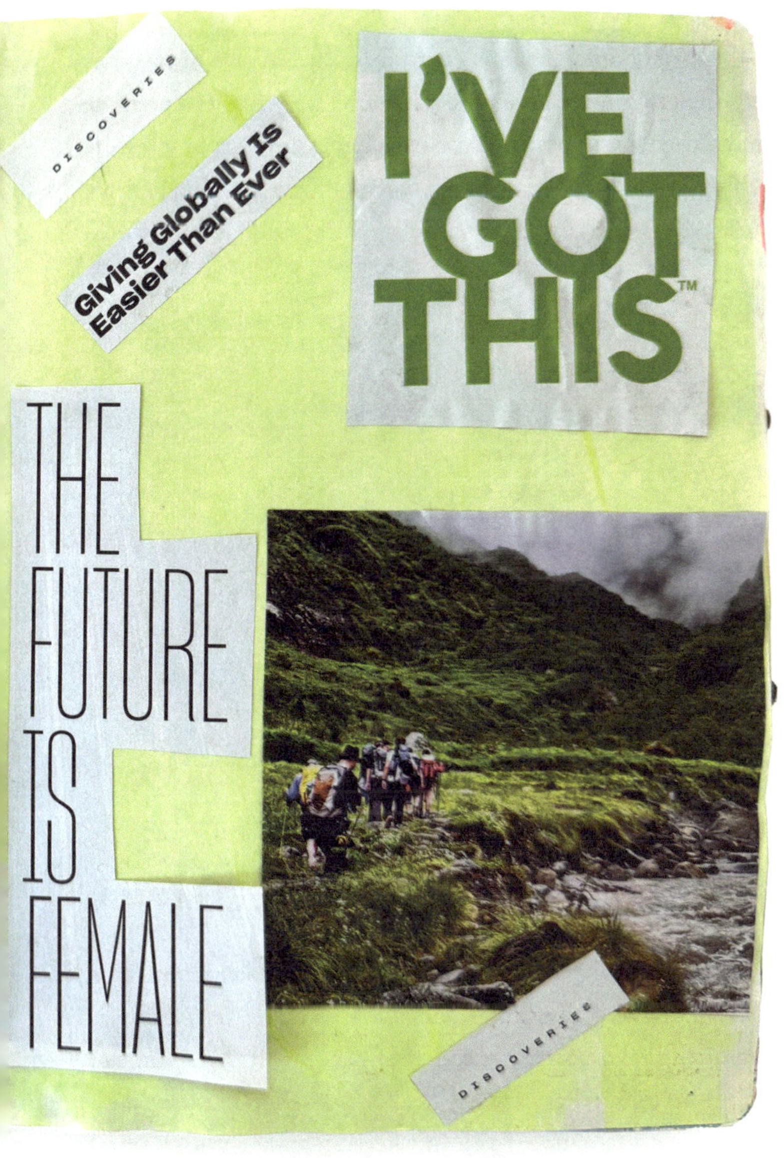

Some entries may be focused on reflections of the past. Some on the state of things today. And others may project the future and allow you to dream.

places we can't always foresee and deal with the surprises and challenges that life hands us, making course adjustments we never could have imagined.

In the same quote, Abrams goes on to say, "As we grow older we cover the ground we have covered before, only higher up; as we look down the winding stair below us, we measure our progress by the number of places where we were but no longer are. The journey is both repetitious and progressive; we go both round and upward."

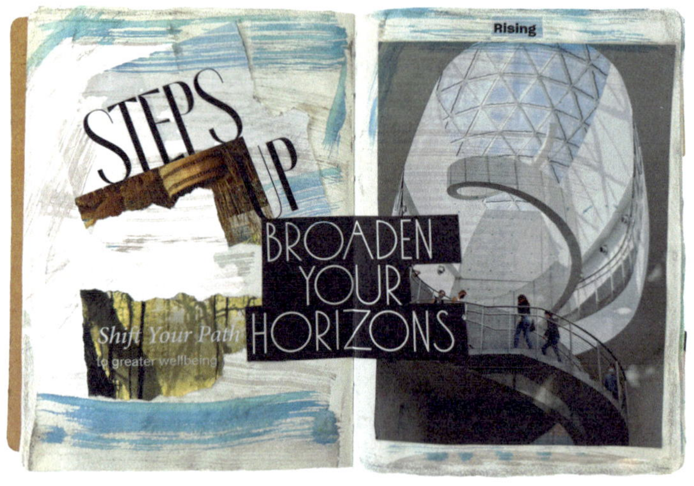

My inner child (voice) encouraging me to keep an open mind. Shapes can inspire thoughts, ideas, and memories too. Triangles, spirals, or circles can provoke different feelings depending on your sense of the world in one moment versus another.

So, life has its inevitable hiccups, missed opportunities, false starts, late starts, and non-starts, but if we view life transitions as curves in our spiral staircase, we can be at peace with the unknown. You might not know what's around the bend, but you can have faith that you'll get to that curve if you just keep stepping. With a spiral staircase, it's the twist and sideways motion that keep us going up. And, as Abrams says, as we progress upward, we're blessed with the ability to look down on the rungs below us, discovering their patterns and learning from them. Maybe the beauty of life *is* the side-to-side movement, the circling back and seeing not only how far we've come but the patterns, steps, and twists that got us to where we are now.

Similarly, art journaling allows you to document what you see when you look down your spiral staircase. Reviewing past pages shows that all the curves had a purpose to get us where we are today. So, when we're next faced with a life change, we can trust the process. We can say, "This unknown thing ahead of me isn't a cliff edge. It's just a curve. It's just part of my staircase." And over time, we learn to loosen our grip on the outcome. We start to view the question "How will it turn out?" with curiosity instead of trepidation. We discover that the process is more self-serving than the outcome.

For example, I wrote this book at retirement age, and I can state emphatically that I didn't hang onto expectations about its outcome nearly as tightly as I would've at 25 years old. Art journaling helps us stop kicking and screaming our way between the stages of life and instead become an observer and trust the process. We can use our art journal to identify opportunities for course correction and respond to surprises with calm and curiosity. Because very rarely will success happen the way we think it will. We must learn to embrace uncertainty because it's the uncertainty—the curve in the staircase—that brings us to the next phase of life.

"We are all wonderful, broken wrecks... We're perfect just as these wonderful, beautiful wrecks. That's part of our common humanity. We're all imperfect."

—EMILIO ESTEVEZ

I was in a state of transition and uncertainty as I wrote this book. In the midst of finalizing my decision to retire, I was traveling be-

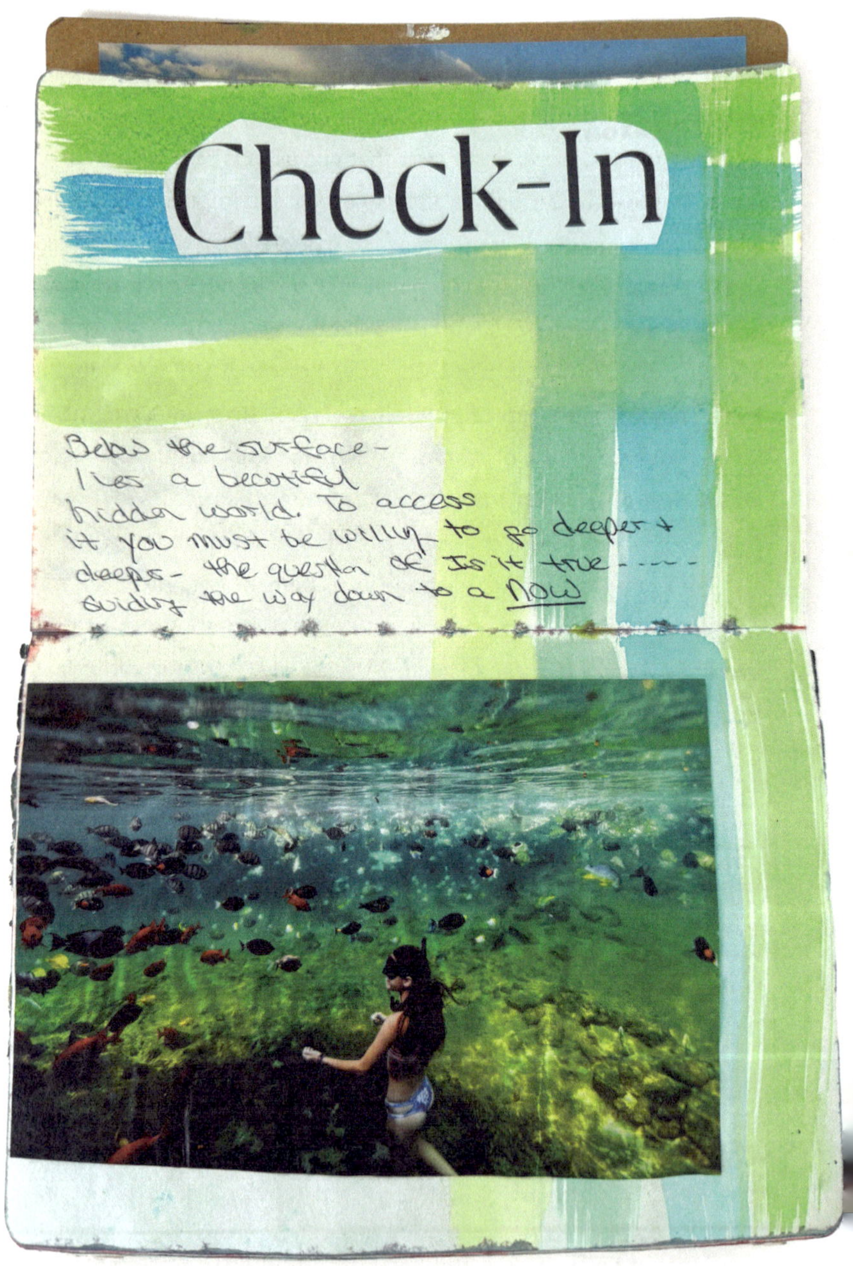

Me reminding myself to check in and go deep.

tween our home in California and our son's in Austin, Texas. My spacious home in California, where my husband and I raised our son, is located in a town that I was moored to for more than 20 years. It's the place I know best; it's where most of my friends and family live. In contrast, the home in Austin is less than 900 square feet total. Still, the cozy home became our refuge during the COVID pandemic, serving as our bright, safe spot during those months of anxiety and uncertainty. I have developed only a smattering of friendships there, but the house in Austin has become like a comfy couch. In time, I will venture out and make new friends. Austin has excellent energy and offers a wide variety of activities; its youthfulness and casualness have been lifelines for me during this transition.

As much as I love both homes, I can't help but feel nomadic at times. My "stuff" is spread out between places. I practically live out of a single roller board and a backpack. The constant transitioning between homes within such a huge life transition (i.e., retirement) often leaves me feeling ungrounded and untethered.

When I feel like that, I remember that home is in me. It's within myself. Home is in my morning routine. It's the song of the birds that greet me each morning I'm in Austin as well as the tweets of the morning birds that greet me in Central Valley of California—different varieties of songs, but morning birdsong nonetheless. Home is the breath of morning air—fresh, dry, and cool in California while thicker and warmer in Austin. Regardless of where I am, the sky never fails to fill with morning light; the trees sway in the imperceptible breeze. I feel like "me" more in the mornings than at any other time of day. But no matter what time of day or what location, I am always at home within myself.

"Cherish sunsets, wild creatures and wild places. Have a love affair with the wonder and beauty of the earth."

—STEWARD AND LEE UDALL

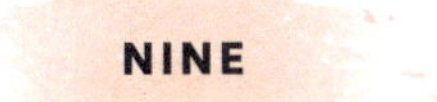

NINE

RETURNING TO YOUR CENTER

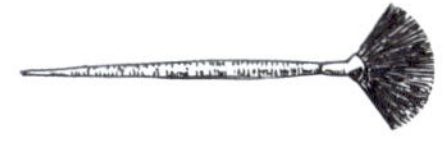

ART JOURNALING ALLOWS YOU TO HAVE A HOME IN YOURSELF, NO MATTER where you are.

I don't really know what I expected retirement to feel like. I have been doing this back-and-forth travel for 18 months now. I would have thought by now that I'd have more of a plan. Sometimes, I try too hard to put one in place and feel the strain of attachment tugging at my happiness level. I release the reins and ask myself, is there actually a problem right now? Usually, the answer is no. Right now, this moment is fantastic, especially if it's a morning moment, with my coffee, with the world slowly waking, with the moon setting and the sun rising.

When I'm having trouble finding this feeling of home within myself, I turn to my art journal, where I find full and deep appreciation for all my blessings. I journal about my gratitude, which reminds me to stay present and unattached to a specific outcome. Journaling brings me home; it eases the urge to push, be productive, and be goal-oriented, helping me to just relish the sheer joy of living.

"Your true home is in the here and the now. It is not limited by time, space, nationality, or race. Your true home is not an abstract idea. It is something you can touch and live in every moment."

—THICH NHAT HANH

I've discovered that it's okay to feel all the highs and lows. In confusing, complex periods of change, we crave clarity—the simple, straightforward, black and white, good or bad. I think that yearning is one of the reasons superhero movies are so popular. It is nice knowing the bad guy is bad and the good guy is good, and of course, it is reassuring to know that good triumphs over evil.

Life, however, is anything but straightforward. In modern society, we enjoy endless options about how we can live, where we live, and what we do with our time. We are freer than ever to challenge what society tells us we "should" be doing during a particular life stage.

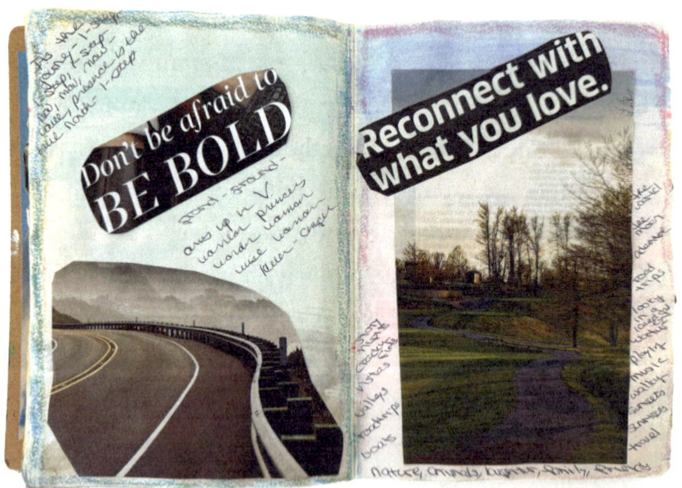

If certain images soothe or inspire you, create them again and again. As an example, I am drawn to images of winding roads and pathways.

Having such freedom, though, can be challenging. Its lack of clear boundaries can leave us anxious and uncertain.

For that reason, I was filled with anxiety as I headed into my retirement, even though it was an anticipated life transition that I had been preparing for, in some form or another, my entire career.

The transition from the structured sphere of working life into unstructured retirement left me feeling uncertain. I was doubting myself, asking questions like, "Am I doing this retirement thing right?" and "Is it supposed to be this hard?"

Perhaps the most confusing part came from the dueling priorities in my head—I so desperately wanted to be free, but I also wanted to stay with the familiar and predictable, where I felt safe, competent, and successful.

I struggled for an answer when asked what I would do next with my life, and I balked at the advice articles proclaiming I needed to have that answer before retiring. That constraint simply wasn't possible for me, nor did I necessarily want it to be. I wanted to chart a different path in my retirement. I wanted to pursue my "wild, free, and filled with joy" mantra, but I didn't know what that looked like, which gave me competing feelings.

"For things to reveal themselves to us, we need to be ready to abandon our views about them."

—THICH NHAT HAHN

I turned to my art journal for solace and some much-needed mental space.

As I worked through those feelings in my art journal, I was increasingly drawn to pictures of mirror images, which made me curious about duality. I wanted to explore that concept further, so I pulled out my dictionary and found the definition of duality

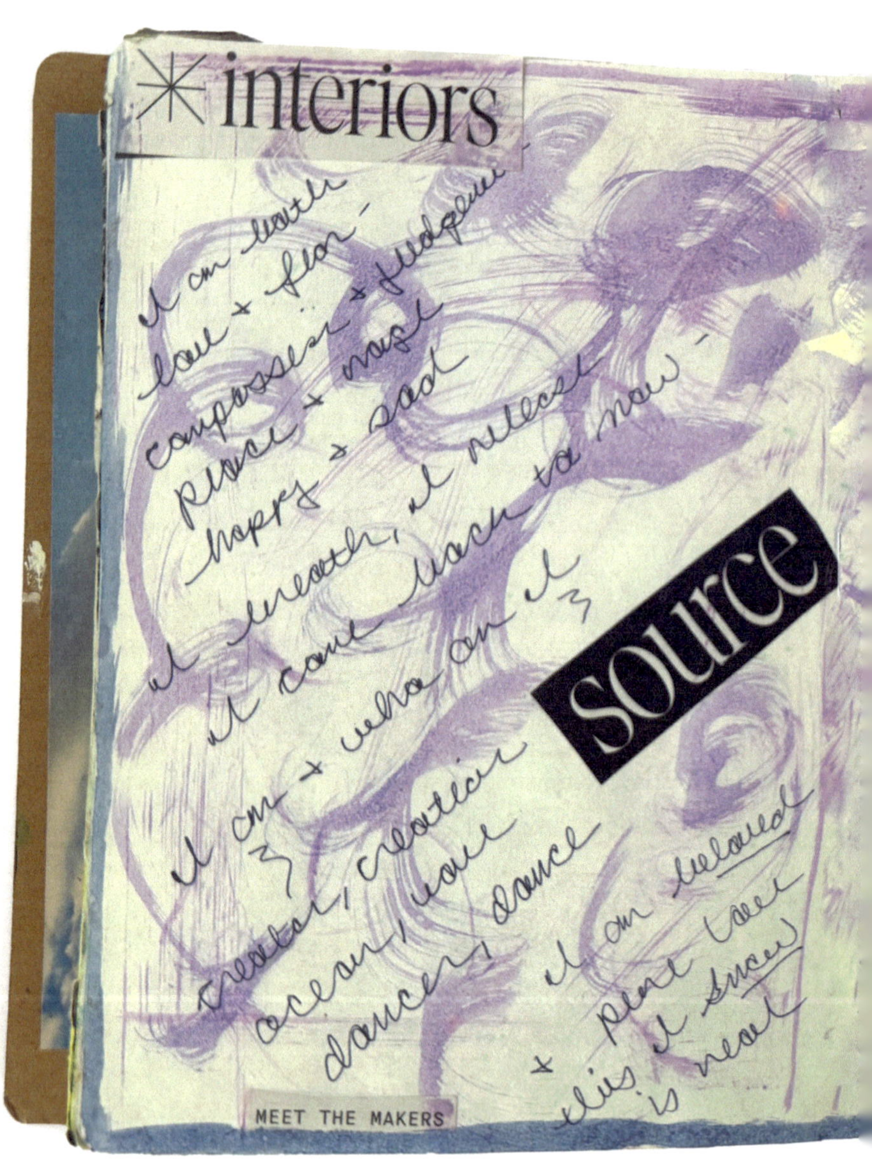
interiors
source
MEET THE MAKERS

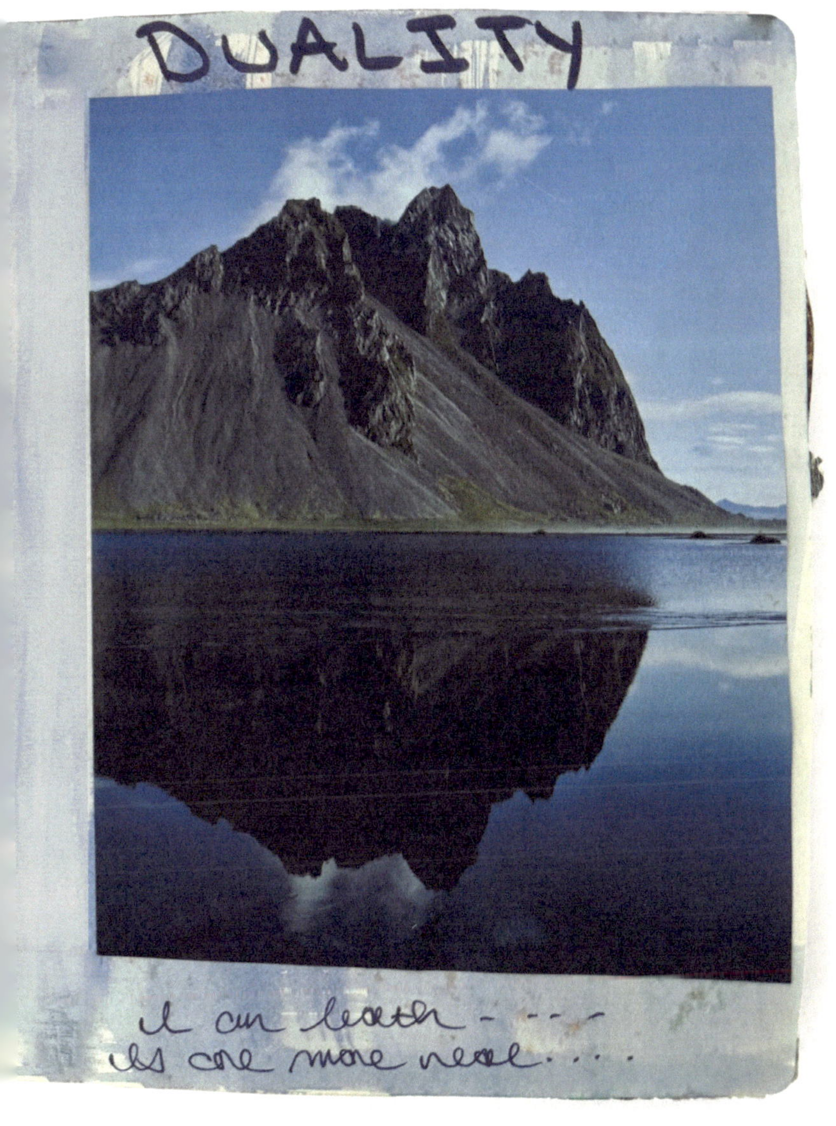

In this image I was playing with duality. Your art journal can become a playground for sorting complex thoughts. Images, charts, and words can help us think forward.

comforting: "Duality refers to having two parts, often with opposite meanings, like the duality of good and evil. If there are two sides to a coin, metaphorically speaking, there's a duality. Peace and war, love and hate, up and down, and black and white are dualities."

I became curious about duality in terms of our thought processes and how we view our world. I'd heard the term "black-and-white thinking" before but had never explored it deeply.

The clinician team at the Trellis Society, a community-development non-profit focused on helping people grow and flourish in all areas of their lives, explained how duality can help us "feel our feelings without getting stuck." In their blog, they explain how embracing duality allows us to shift our thought patterns out of the rigid black-and-white pattern to create space for growth.

I began to wonder if my black-and-white thinking was hindering my transition. Did I really have to have every aspect of my retirement perfectly planned? Yes, I was balking at the societal norm that retirement should be a predesigned event, but it wasn't like I was planning to do nothing but binge-watch TV all day, either.

The term "duality" defined the conflicting emotions I was feeling about retirement. What I found particularly interesting in the Trellis Society's article was the idea that opposing forces in duality (e.g., opposing emotions) don't have to repel one another. Instead, conflicting emotions not only can coexist but even be complementary to one another. When you approach life with the understanding that everything exists on a continuum with opposite extremes at both ends and a murky middle in between, you are better able to find harmony amid uncertainty.

As I worked with duality in my art journal, I was continually struck by the power of color—how using contrasting colors together felt good. It felt real.

The contrasting colors gave life and vivaciousness to the blank page. I realized if colors, no matter how different, can coexist, then maybe my emotions could too. Maybe more than one truth—or one emotion—can simultaneously exist, even if they contradict each other.

I realized that my dueling apprehension and excitement for retirement was okay. It's healthy to feel more than one emotion at one time—all emotions are true simultaneously. I could move myself from the rigidness of either/or thinking through image and color.

Black-and-white thinking can back us into a corner, leaving us emotionally frustrated and confused. Art journaling can help us move from requiring ourselves to feel "this *or* that" emotion to accepting that we feel "this *and* that" and that duality of emotion is not only normal but healthy. As I worked with these challenging, dueling emotions, I was continuously delighted by what appeared on the pages of my art journal. I felt "seen" by some of my most conflicted pages. I came to appreciate the continuum of feelings that sprang to life in the pages of my journal.

> *"Do I contradict myself?*
> *Very well then I contradict myself,*
> *(I am large, I contain multitudes)."*
>
> —WALT WHITMAN

TEN

LETTING GO OF FEAR TO CHOOSE GROWTH

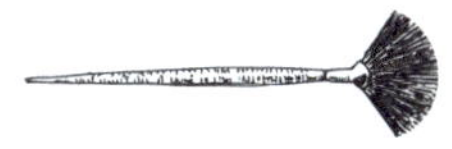

FEAR IS THE MOST COMMON EMOTION ASSOCIATED WITH CHANGE. THERE'S actually a dedicated word for "fear of change": *metathesiophobia.* Above all other emotions, fear is probably the one that makes it most challenging to pursue our goals or make positive changes to our lives. But it's hard to rid ourselves of fear, especially when we're facing a big transition in life, because fear is a normal emotion. We even have a part of our brain, the amygdala, that's dedicated to fear-based processing. So being fearful of change is hardwired into our neurocircuitry. Nevertheless, it's better to accept the fear instead of trying to push it out with faith. That action actually tends to make us avoidant, anxious, and pretty darn miserable altogether. The key is to make just as much room for your fear as you do for your faith. Art journaling can help you get to build a more adaptable mindset that embraces change and the fear that comes along with it.

"One can choose to go back toward safety or forward toward growth. Growth must be chosen again and again: fear must be overcome again and again."

—ATTRIBUTED TO ABRAHAM MASLOW

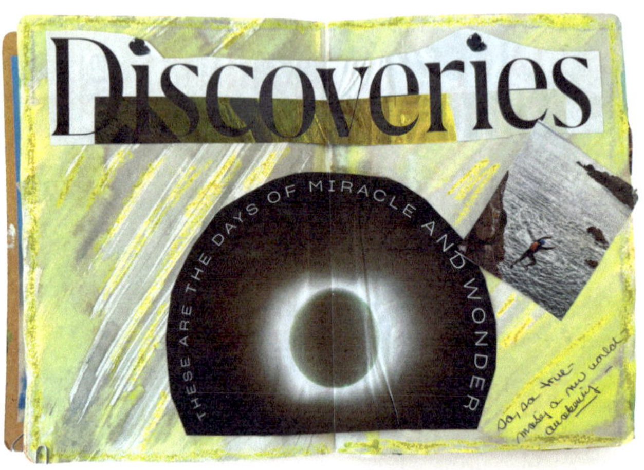

When you notice a pattern of recurring images that are inspiring or even disturbing, your art journal is a safe place to explore this. For example, I found lots of images of people jumping off cliffs during this time in my life, and my art journal helped me to put the idea of gutsy jumps in a more joyful context.

Sometimes, we just don't know how to move forward, period. In those cases, I like to follow Harvard-trained sociologist and world-renowned life coach and author Martha Beck's advice when it feels as though everything is changing and no one knows what is coming next. She says:

> There are two parts of you that know. Call them the eagle and the mouse. The eagle can rise up high and see your whole life. It sees where you've been. It sees where you can go. Connect with it by asking: 'How do I want the world to be different because I

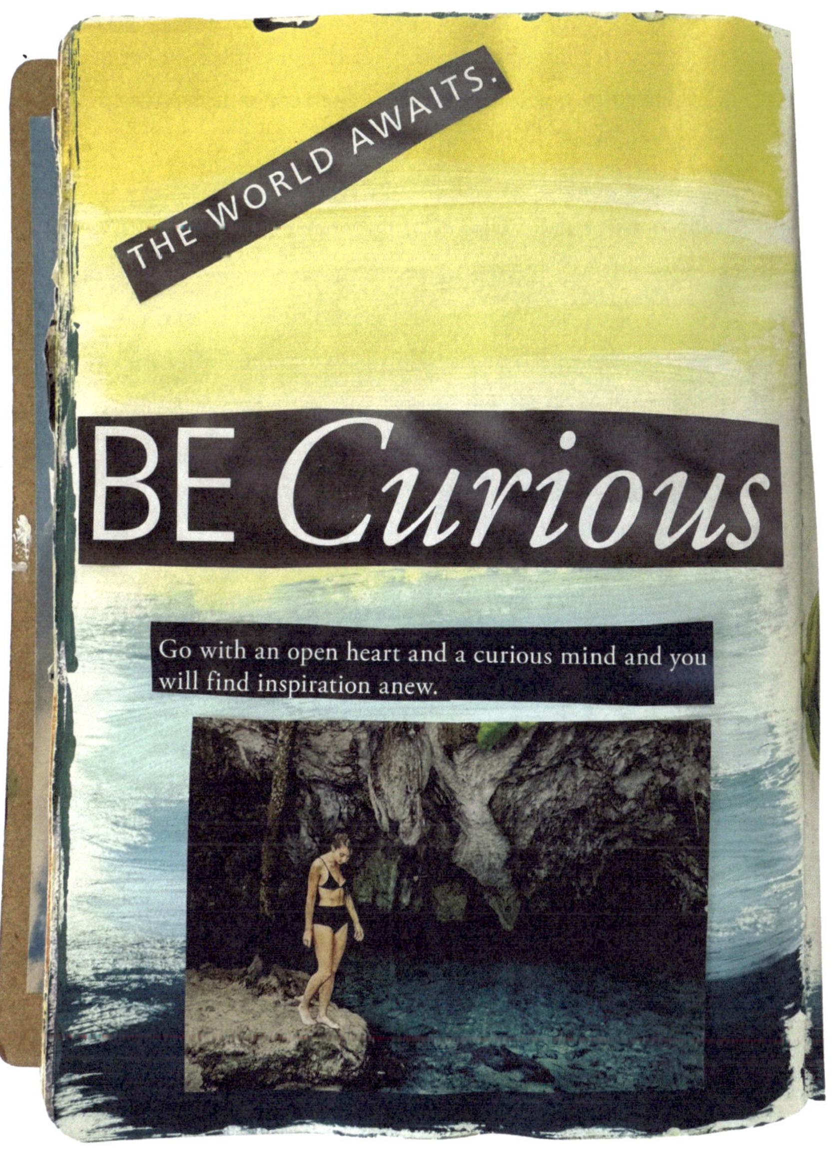

When a thought crystallizes, a simple, bold art journal entry becomes a powerful talisman to keep that idea front and center for you. This one says it all.

> have lived?' Once you see that goal with your eagle eyes, write it down. Mark that spot on the horizon. Now become your mouse self. It can't see far, but it knows what's right in front of you. Ask it, 'What's the smallest step I can take now to move me toward my eagle vision?'

Both are valid viewpoints, and each has its place. The eagle-eye view gives us a broad picture of where we want to go—it lays out a map in front of us. While maps are helpful, their broad dimensions can be overwhelming. That situation is where the mouse comes in. The mouse can't see that whole map; he only sees what is just in front of him. He asks himself, "What is the next smallest step I can take?" That mindset can be fostered through art journaling by asking ourselves the same question. Exploring the question via the journal page can bring a lot of insight. Then you can take your "smallest next step" and view it in the context of your eagle-eye map (which you could also journal on, by the way). The idea is to continuously move yourself back and forth between eagle and mouse mindsets to make sure you remain aligned during your transition.

The perspectives of the eagle and the mouse can show a path toward the future, but they don't expose our fears, which tend to impede forward movement. I see art journaling as a way to reveal our fears—the logical, linear thoughts about fear encompassing the what ifs, worst-case scenarios, and images of abject failure—and move them from the left brain to the right brain. In the right brain, scary linear thoughts transform into benign symbols, and there's space for play and possibility. Letting the right brain lead is an excellent tool to open you up or create some curiosity. Colors and images will move you from the constricts of fear because the fear in what comes next is a function of your left brain and the discernment of thinking.

With the constraints of fear reduced—if not removed—we can

explore what is possible on the blank page before us, using color and shape, or even quotes, collages, or anything else, really. Art journaling is a way to move out of a loop that is blocking you. It's almost like being willing to take a detour, and on that detour, you might just discover faith, confidence, and joy.

"The only way to make sense out of change is to plunge into it, move with it, and join the dance."

—ALAN WATTS

Take a moment to write down your fears. What comes up in your body when you allow yourself to think those thoughts? Sure, it's uncomfortable, but just feel them. Breathe into them. Take three, deep, slow breaths.

What colors or images come up for you when you look at your fears as an observer. Choose one fear, maybe not the worst, scariest one, but a medium one to start and color it. Release it onto the page in whatever form you like. How does it look? What colors, textures, words, or images go with it?

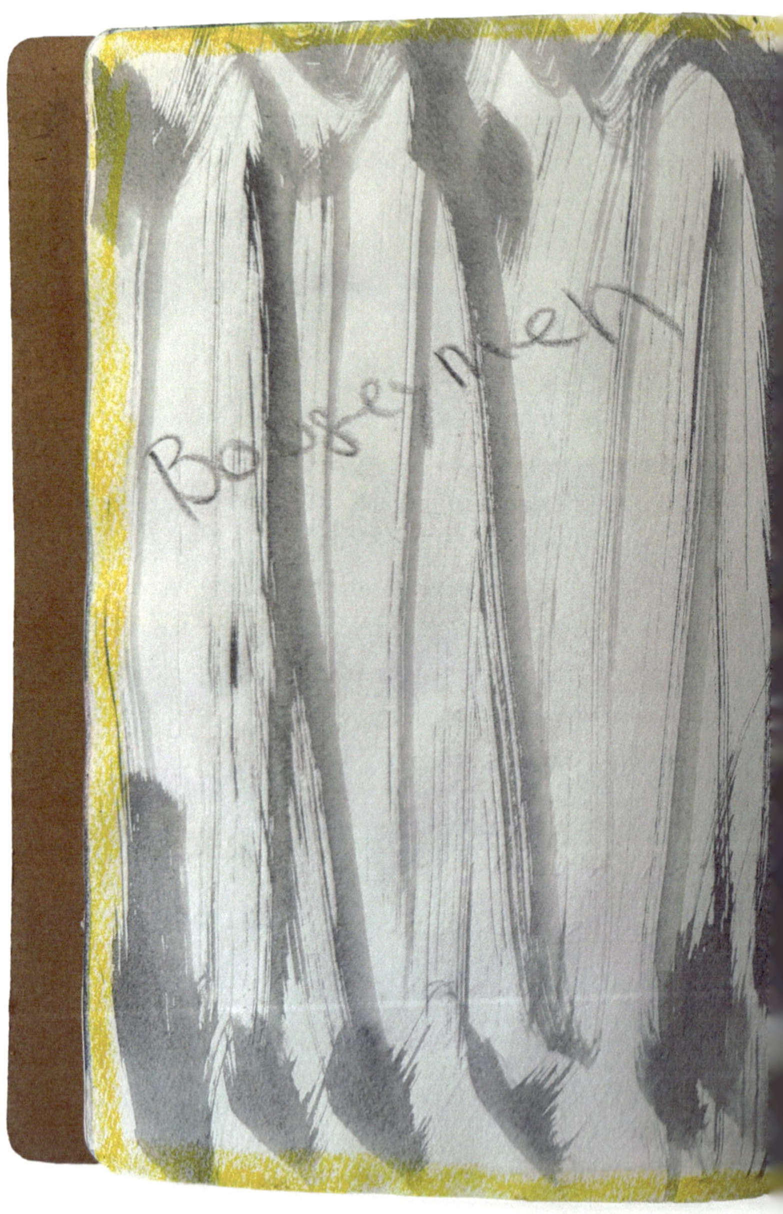
Bogeymen

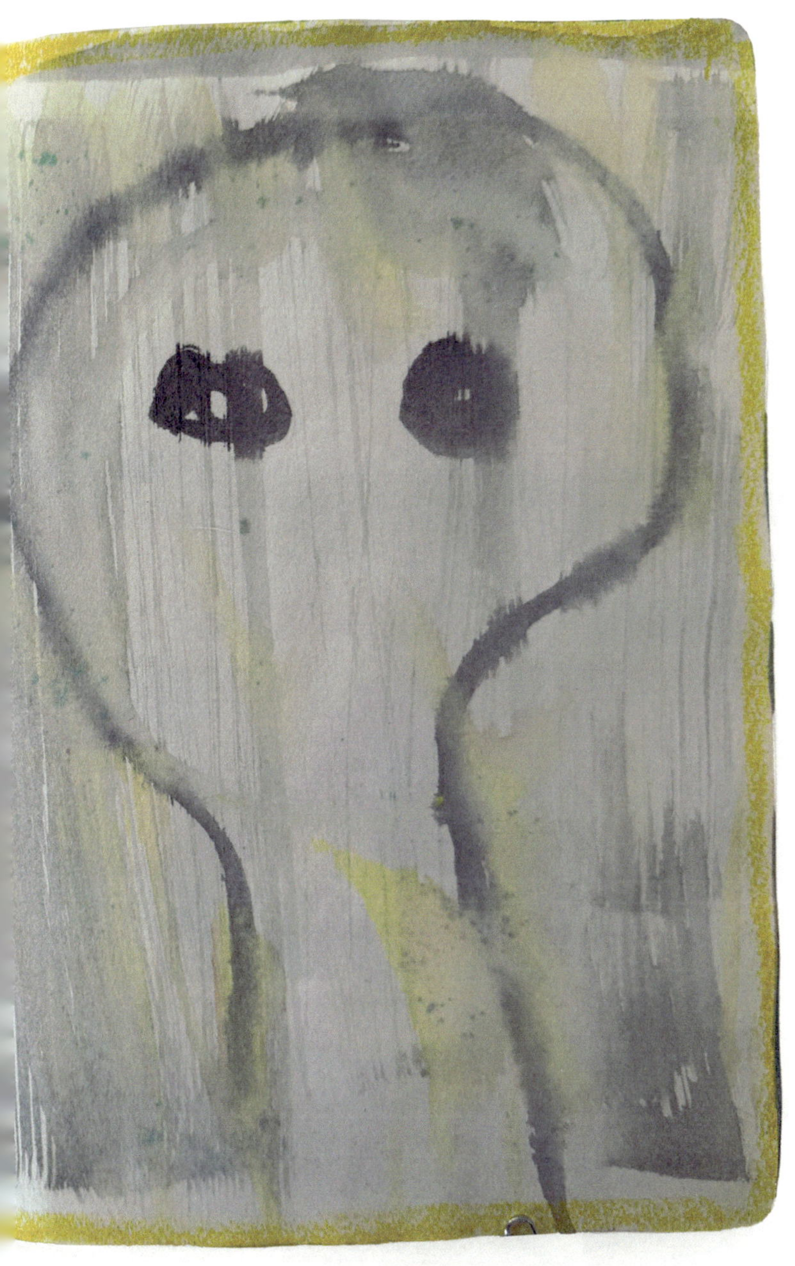

Facing your fear by expressing it on paper. My boogeyman.

Part Four

A SAFE PLACE

Art journaling is a safe way to explore our full range of emotions.

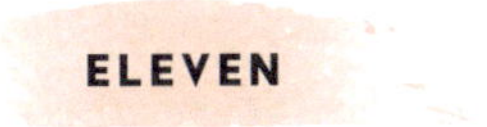

ELEVEN

WHEN LIFE KNOCKS YOU DOWN

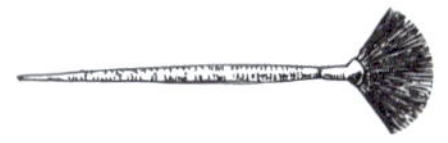

WHEN LIFE IS A BULLY, MOST PEOPLE RETREAT, WHICH IS A NATURAL reaction. Hurt feelings need space and solace to recover our dignity after being upset by others. I propose art journaling as safe way to explore our full range of emotions—happy or hurt.

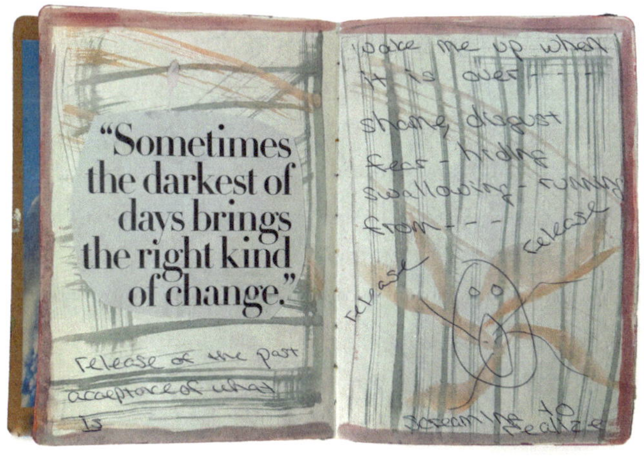

An art journal is a place to express extreme emotions. In this case, mine became a holding place for my screams.

Bullies are all around us, unfortunately. Sometimes, life itself can be a bully; life circumstances that are outside of our control can bring us to our knees as if we were at the mercy of a bully on the playground. Succumbing to those effects can rob us of our innocence, awe, and sense of wonder. Indeed, the scars of life's bullying often are deep and long-lasting. But surviving and working through such experiences can make you a stronger, kinder, and more confident person. And that's the secret.

"A day came when the risk to remain tight in a bud was more painful than the risk it took to blossom."

—ELIZABETH APPELL

Here's my story. I had dreamed of being a journalist since the sixth grade when I won a county-wide essay contest. My essay, titled "Happy Birthday Uncle Sam," earned me a $200 savings bond and my picture in the local newspaper. From that moment on, when asked what I wanted to be when I grew up, I would say a writer. But looking back, I think my dream job would be better described as a communicator because writer eventually turned into journalist into reporter.

I remember being captivated by the news while riding the stationary bike in our family room. It was during the hostage crisis in Iran, the era when *Nightline* was born. The news at the time was particularly important; dreaming about being able to share it was exhilarating. I wanted to be on it—the news, not the bike. It seemed to me that there could be no greater calling than bringing information to people. I believed that helping to show what was happening could be my contribution to the world.

As soon as I could, I started to get internships in newsrooms in the Bay Area. Then I earned a master's degree in journalism, followed by my first job as a TV journalist.

I was so thrilled to be promoted from journalist to main anchor-producer. I was just 24 years old! I loved every aspect of my job, and I was marinating in the sense that my dreams were being fulfilled.

That is until I was bullied at work. I started to receive anonymous notes inside my desk drawer, outlining any mistake I had made during a newscast the night before and telling me to go back to my previous news station. Because the notes were anonymous, I didn't know whom to trust. Was it just one person? Or were several of my coworkers in on it?

Those incidents took the wind out of my sails, as only bullying can. The innocence and awe in me died. As I reflect, the shock of being bullied was worse than what they said or did. It was the shock of becoming the object of someone else's meanness, of the smallness I felt, and of the feeling of being misunderstood and abandoned by my coworkers whom I thought of as friends.

I was hurt deeply, but I would emerge a stronger, kinder, more confident woman. After due reflection, I came to a deeper understanding that the bullying nature of my coworkers was a reflection of their insecurity, not of my shortcomings. After that realization found its place in my heart and mind, I was able to look at my bullies with a level of both dispassion and compassion. After all, for them, it was easier to be mean. It was easier to tear someone else down than to lift themselves up, which would make them vulnerable to the very rejection they dished out to me. Their rejection left me with nothing to lose, and I realized that I wouldn't crumble and I wouldn't fall apart. I would keep going.

If you're in those shoes, look to art journaling as a way to take back your innocence, awe, and sense of wonder. It provides a safe place to vent and to heal. Turning to my art journal in times of emotional turmoil is like turning into the arms of the truest and sincerest of friends. It's always ready to listen and help me process even the most difficult of emotions.

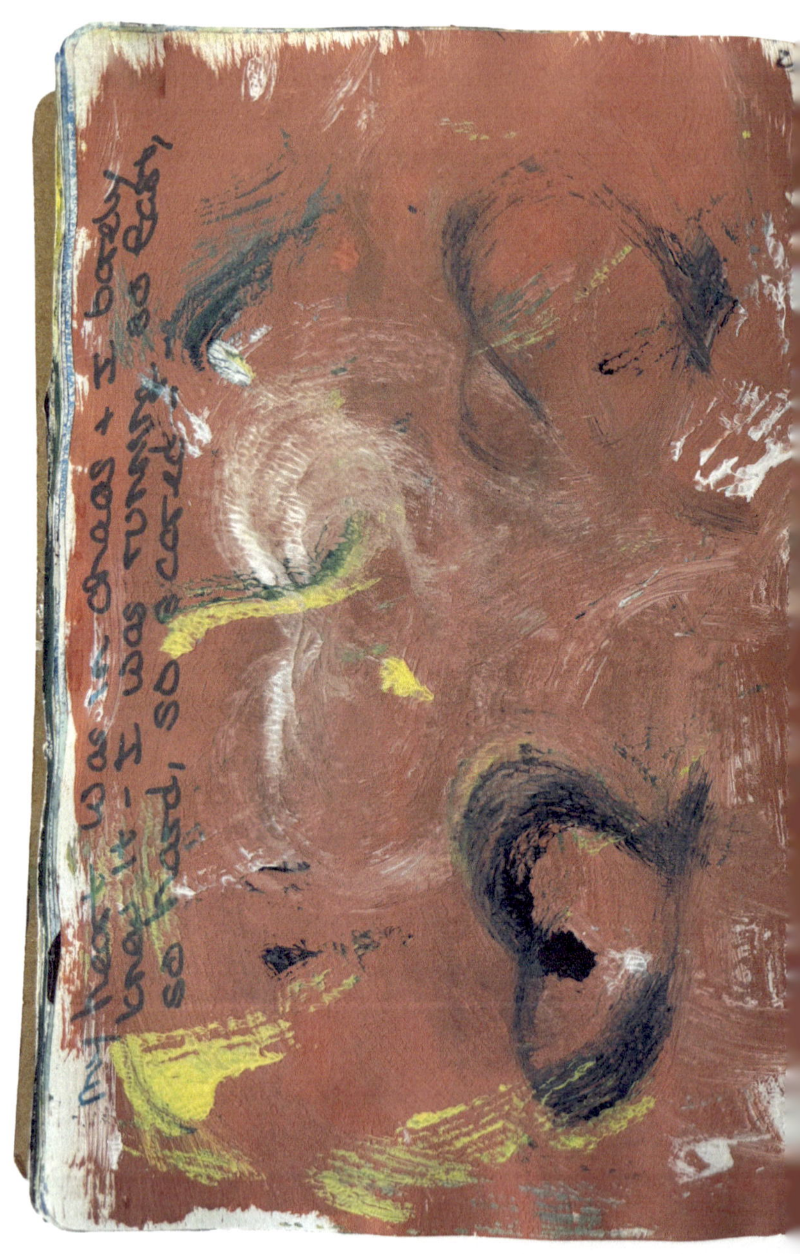
My heart was in chaos + I barely
knew it - I was running so fast,
so hard, so scared, so sad,

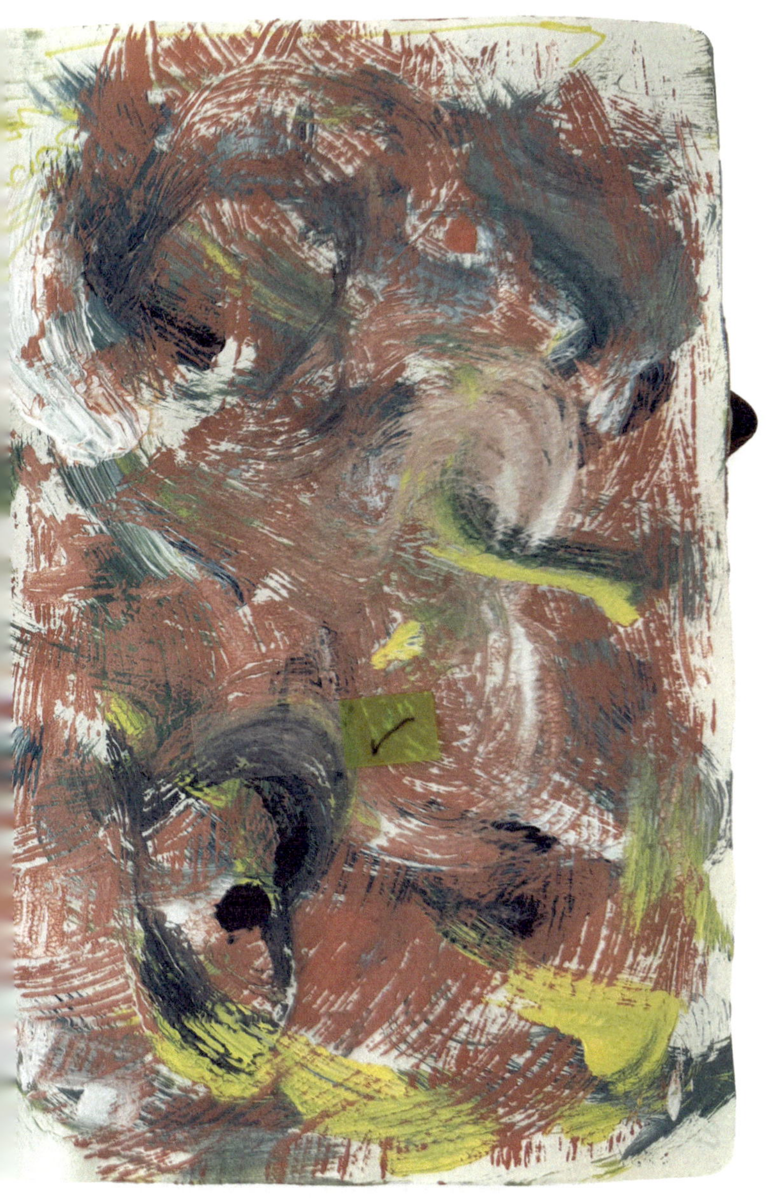

Capturing the chaos in my heart.

TWELVE

THE HEALING EFFECTS OF ART JOURNALING

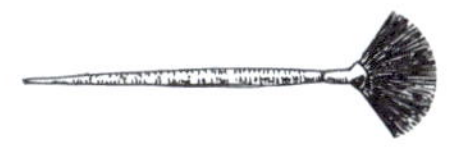

HAVE YOU EVER BEEN FEELING DOWN OR UPSET AND COULDN'T REALLY put your finger on what emotion you were feeling and why? Neurobiologists have found that some negative emotions—especially grief or trauma—are processed in a part of our brain that can't be accessed verbally or even consciously. Their discovery means that our emotions sometimes can be the type that we literally "have no words for" and can't "wrap our minds around," so to speak. Sometimes, I myself find that I feel stuck in an emotion, and I've learned that my art journal is the best "listener" in those cases. The act of art journaling frees me from the constraints of language, which allows me to explore feelings that otherwise might be difficult to articulate or even think about. (An added bonus is that it frees me from the fear of judgment, criticism, or rejection.)

I've also found that art journaling seems to take me out of my logical brain left brain—the area of the brain that thinks in a structured and linear fashion—and moves me into the right side of the brain, where I'm able to process things more easily.

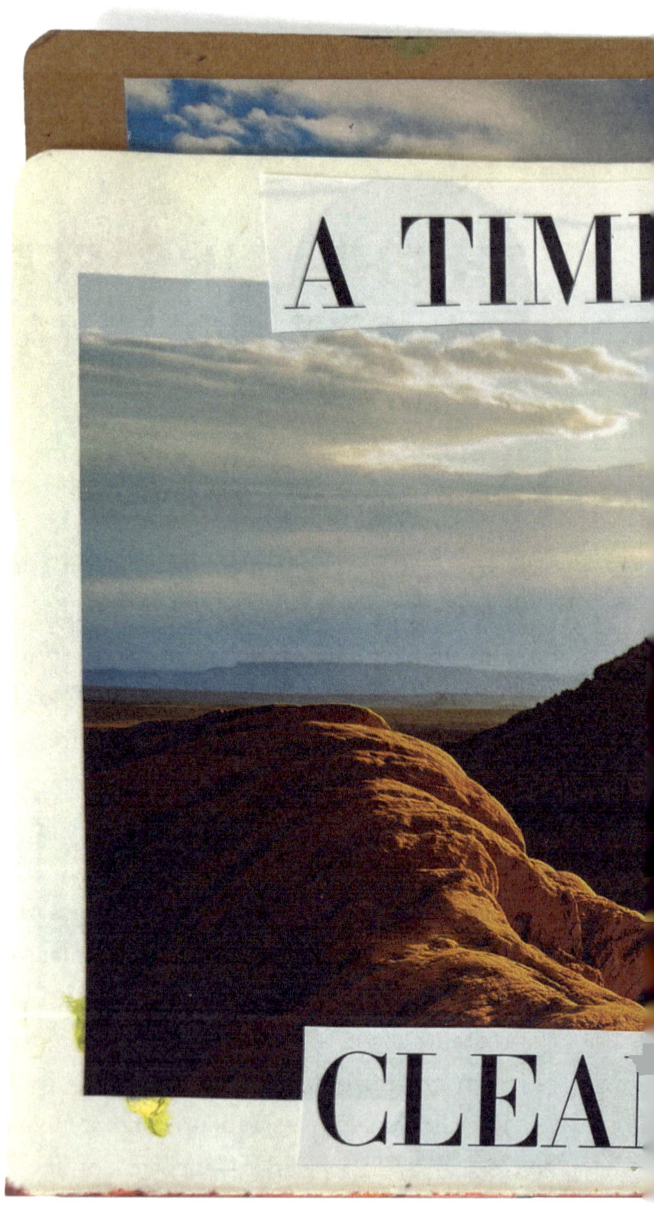
A TIM
CLEA

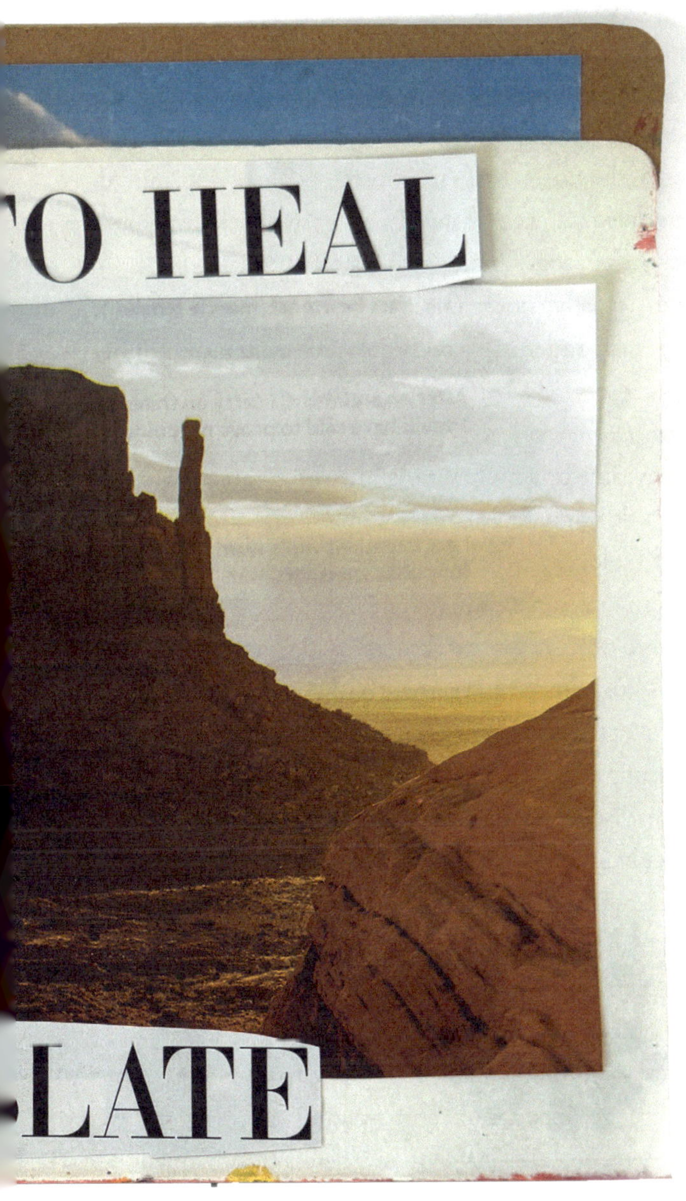

Use your art journal as a place to express your pain and begin to heal.

Neuroanatomist Jill Bolte Taylor, PhD, has an explanation for why this "switch" might be the case. Dr. Taylor worked at Harvard in neurosciences, studying how brains create our perception of reality when she tragically became a subject of her own research at age 37: She survived a massive stroke in which the left side of her brain shut down. This shift altered the entire way she operated—how she moved, spoke, and responded. It even changed her sense of self-awareness. Since that time, she's become an impactful speaker, sharing powerful ways that we can actually choose our state of mind. We can replace feelings of stress, fear, and anxiety with those of joy and deep inner peace. You can read more in her book *My Stroke of Insight: A Brain Scientist's Personal Journey*, but to summarize, she shares how we can calm ourselves any time by simply tuning into the inherent peacefulness of the right side of the brain.

In her book, Taylor says, "Peace is only a thought away." At first, the statement sounded super-esoteric and impractical at best, but then she went on to explain. Her stroke impacted almost the entirety of her left brain—just shut it down completely. To compensate, the right brain took over the entirety of her cognitive processing (isn't the human body absolutely incredible?). Interestingly, after her stroke happened, Taylor discovered she felt different. To her surprise, she felt calm and totally in touch with the world. She was neither scared about the present nor fearful for the future. She felt mindful and at peace. The shift made her look at things differently. If that state of mindfulness was achieved by effectively the shutting down her left brain, then that outcome means that these feelings of peace, wholeness, and calm are within us all along. Simply stated, we don't *create* these feelings through meditation and mindfulness exercises; we simply *uncover* them. We all innately have these amazing qualities. They're there, just waiting for us to uncover them, and it's exactly what she meant by "peace is only a thought away."

In my experience, art journaling gives us a direct connection to our right brain. We can access that connection any time by carrying our journal around with us or storing it in a handy place in the house. It's powerful.

We don't need to spend hours in meditation, pay for expensive yoga classes, or read dozens of books on mindfulness. A fresh art journaling page is always there, ready to help when we're in need of an emotional breather or a reality check.

"There's almost no such thing as ready. There's only now."

—HUGH LAURIE

Think of your art journal as a container for your thoughts and emotions. Each of us needs to find a place to hold our difficult emotions. They are painful and difficult to process, but leaving them uncontained allows them to resurface continually and cause us anxiety or worse. Emotions that are overwhelming and tumultuous usually trigger our fear response, as if facing them will make us capsize or fall overboard. At such times, I turn to art journaling because it has a knack for bottling that storm of emotions into a tidy container through which I can observe my thoughts and feelings with curiosity and detachment—without getting swept away by them.

In that way, art journaling is actually very similar to meditation. However, wonderful as it is, meditation can be really challenging at times. Although I have meditated daily for years, I found art journaling to be a terrific complement to meditation, as is traditional journaling. With meditation, the container that holds our thoughts and emotions ebbs and flows in and out of reach. Access to it is dependent on our ability to practice mindful awareness in the moment. I don't know about you, but this isn't always easy for me. Sometimes, meditation can be too esoteric and ephemeral for me.

Art journaling is much more straightforward than meditation, and you're rewarded with the same result. Unlike meditation, art journaling presents our thoughts and feelings as tangible ideas—we can see them right there in front of us. The page of the art journal is the container. And that page is there no matter what state I'm in—mindful or otherwise. As a convenient container, it displays our thoughts and emotions, which take on the forms of color and shape, presenting themselves within collages or in some cases, actual words and phrases.

The innumerable shades of a color palette and a wide range of media provide an instant source in order to capture our feelings. I use color quite a bit in my art journal to help me process difficult emotions. And, wow, does it help! I'm not surprised that researchers have found that coloring reduces stress and anxiety. They say it also increases relaxation, which I have definitely found the case to be true for me. I think it's particularly interesting (and also unsurprising) that unstructured coloring activities were found to have the most profound impact on stress and anxiety, as opposed to more structured art activities.

Researchers aren't sure yet exactly how or why that effect works, other than the idea that art can diminish activity in the fear portion of our brain. I know for me, art journaling works to do all those things and much more, which is all the evidence that I need.

In art therapy, practitioners use color to improve mood. Basically, each color on the visible color spectrum (i.e., red, orange, yellow, green, blue, indigo, and violet) vibrates at a different frequency, and using a specific color will shift the energy and frequencies within our bodies to match that vibration.

That effect is true in my case, that's for sure. For example, I particularly love pink and yellow. When I see pink or yellow on my page, it just instantly makes me feel super happy, even if I've been crazy stressed all day. I don't need to know the science behind it as much as I just need to know it works for me.

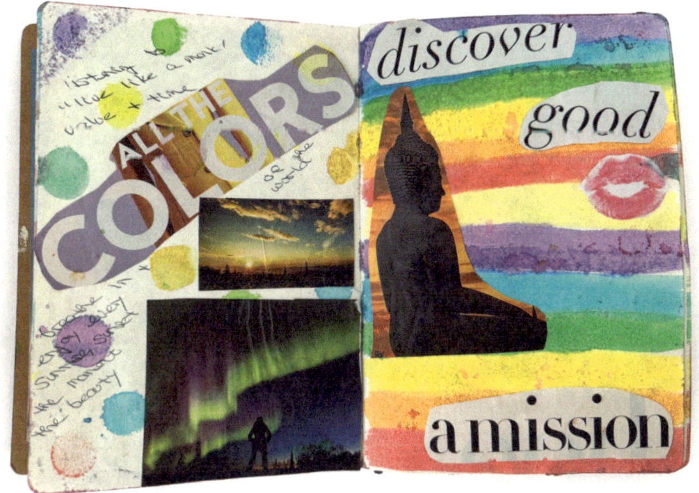

Loving all the colors, accepting all emotions. You can use color to serve as a starting point to represent the array of emotions that you're currently experiencing.

On some days, the red, blue, and violet colors appeal to me more if I'm upset or worried about some matter. Through my art journaling, those colors give sense to my feelings, assuage my emotions, and are particularly effective in turning what seem like scary monsters into grazing sheep. The hues remind me of one of my favorite children's books, *Where the Wild Things Are* by Maurice Sendak. My favorite line was "The wild things roared their terrible roars and gnashed their terrible teeth and rolled their terrible eyes and showed their terrible claws, but Max stepped into his private boat and waved goodbye."

At the end of the story Max realizes he can have wild feelings in all their glory, but that his mom will still love him and all his big feelings no matter what. That realization helps him to ultimately re-center himself.

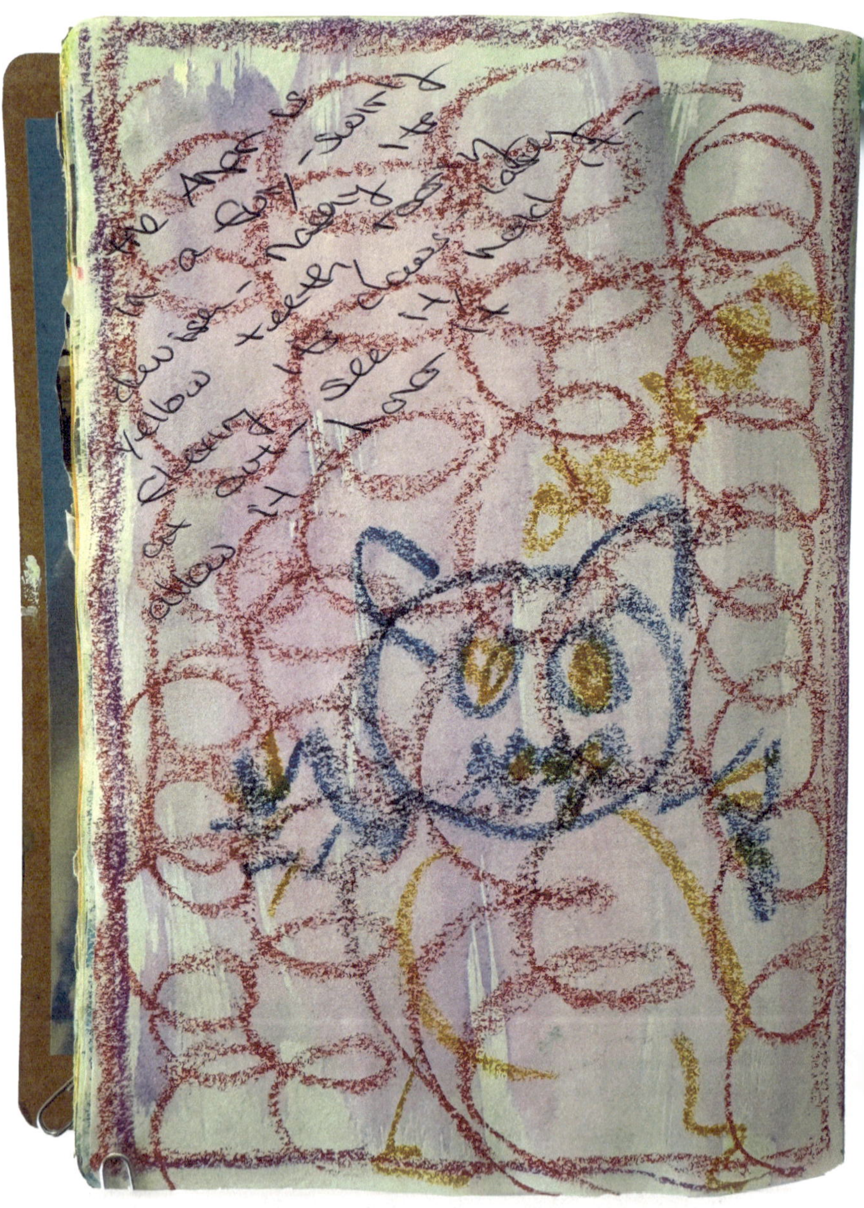

My wild thing.

Likewise, my art journal has served as a place where I can let my anger roar its terrible roar and gnash its terrible teeth in a safe place, a place that is actually fun to look back upon, a place where I am not apologizing for something I said in a fit of anger, a place where I can get centered and figure out the next right thing to say or do. In my experience there is never a next right thing to do when my blood is boiling.

In fact, one of my favorite entries in my art journal is a wild thing I drew in crayon. It's only my four-year-old-artist version that makes it look like one of the wild things from Sendak's beautifully illustrated book, but with a dark blue crayon I created a screaming wild thing, with slashing claws, and lots of red. As I drew, I was able to express the swirling anger in my large red swirls. As the emotions relaxed, my anger started to dissipate. Just at that moment, I could watch it, honor it, give it a face, teeth, claws. It felt like a swirling dervish, the words from Sendak's book playing in my head.

When I was done, I felt good, composed. I could then find the right course of action, the right words that would honor my boundaries and speak a calm truth. The picture helped to create a space so that I could have a conversation that would honor the situation when I was centered and at peace, and best yet, there was no apology needed because I sought to use my art journal before acting. Even to this day, I love my angry wild thing.

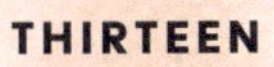

THIRTEEN

LABELING DIFFICULT EMOTIONS

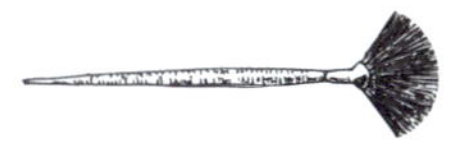

"The limits of my language mean the limits of my world."

—LUDWIG WITTGENSTEIN

WHEN I FEEL A NEGATIVE EMOTION, I FIND A HELPFUL FIRST STEP IS TO LABEL that emotion. Labeling can be tricky, though, right? It's one thing to say, "I'm angry," but it's a little more difficult to elaborate. Do I actually mean it to be something else? Disappointed, jealous, hurt, frustrated, sad, or perhaps just confused? The differences between those descriptors may seem minute, but using language to differentiate and label an emotion is vital to working through it.

In her book *Atlas of the Heart*, Brené Brown, PhD, MSW, says, "Language is our portal to meaning-making, connection, healing, learning, and self-awareness. Having access to the right words can open up entire universes...Language shows us that naming an experience doesn't give the experience more power, it gives us the power of understanding and meaning."

Art journaling has helped me understand the deeper roots of my emotions, especially when I felt angry. Before I used art journaling, I assumed I was an angry person because I felt "anger" often. But art journaling has helped me to go deeper and uncover what my "anger" really was. Through the shapes and colors on the page, I began to intuitively see what was really happening inside me. The picture didn't always offer immediate clarification, but as the paint dried or the collage took shape, I could see that my anger wasn't actually anger at all. The real emotions were sadness, fear, and hurt, which can physically feel like anger and even mentally sound like it. But they're so different from anger, right? Before art journaling, my insistence on the idea that I was angry was keeping me from addressing the fact that I felt small, vulnerable, and alone. It's a bit ironic that by allowing my four-year-old artist to first release these emotions onto the page using color, shapes, and paints, I could finally understand that I was secure and safe. Labeling my feeling of "anger" by its true name dissolved its power over me.

Your art journal can be a map of your emotions, feelings, and state of mind. Here are a few ways to use your art journal to label your emotions. I used Brené Brown's book *Atlas of the Heart* as a guide. Try picking a statement below and begin to use your art journal to see if the statement changes.

"I feel overwhelmed."

Do you actually feel stress, anxiety, worry, avoidance, excitement, dread, fear, vulnerability, or something else?

"I feel disappointed."

Do you actually feel bored, regretful, discouraged, resigned, or frustrated?

"I feel hurt."

Do you actually feel anguish, hopelessness, despair, sadness, or grief?

You get the idea.

Grief
what grows beneath
the tears
+ heartbreak?
love
both old + new
changed -> transformed

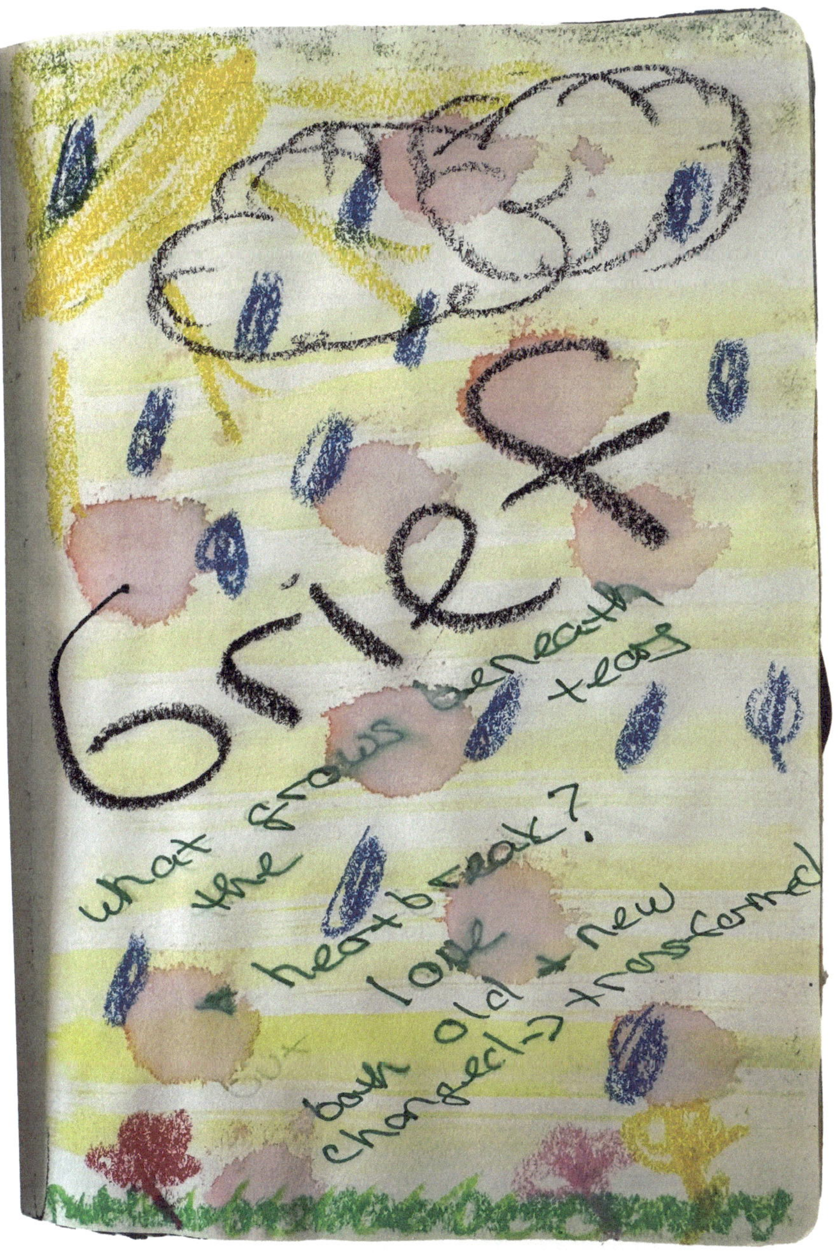

Grief.

Now take a moment to think of some of the most recent emotions that have been cycling through you in the last few days. Write them down, then choose one and start playing with what it looks like in color or image. As you play, don't be afraid to add words or capture thoughts along with the colors and images.

After a few minutes, take a few breaths, step back, and admire what your inner artist has unleashed! Then keep adding on if it feels good, or start a new page with a new emotion.

Many times, I have several pages going at once, and as emotions soften or change, I keep adding to the page. I like to draw crayon borders on my pages, which give me the feeling that I am creating a safe place for the emotion to come to full expression.

Part Five

A PATH TO SELF-DISCOVERY

Art journaling allows us to uncover clues to our heart's desires.

FOURTEEN

ENJOY THE JOURNEY

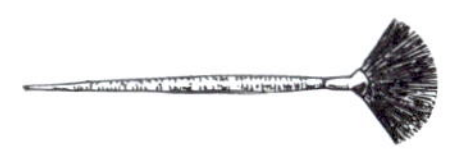

AS AN ADULT, I'VE WORKED WITH THERAPISTS, SERVED AS A COACH DURING my HR career, explored yoga, traditional journaling, and meditation—the works. So, it's safe to say that I've been thoroughly "tuned up" over the years regarding my personal awareness. Each modality has been helpful in its own right, but art journaling is different: It accesses a part of myself that other ways or things couldn't.

Now, whether it's the art journaling alone or my particular circumstances that are so effective, I can't say. But I can confidently tell you that my art journal has helped me to deeply internalize truths that have been right in front of me all along.

For example, take the saying, "enjoy the journey." It's everywhere in our culture, right? I mean, look in any Target and you'll probably find a mug or T-shirt with "enjoy the journey" in boldface across the front. I feel it's such a shame that the sheer amount of nonstop exposure to well-meaning statements like these turns them into clichés. We're numb to their valuable messages because we see them, hear them—and even say them—all the time.

Art journaling changed that impression for me. Clearly, I could understand what "enjoy the journey" meant at the intellectual level—the mind level—but couldn't quite seem to internalize it at the heart level. What did those words mean to me, to my life? And, even more so, what should I do with them? It's like I was numb to the truth carried in the message. But my art journal opened my heart's receptivity to their true meaning, helping me to understand what its message truly meant to me and how I could authentically apply it to my life.

It started with the word "journey," which led me to use collages, colors, and shapes to reflect on the many journeys I've walked through to get to where I am today. One stood out in particular: the period of my life when I was raising my child. Haven't we all had that period of life when we felt we were the best versions of ourselves? I've always thought that I was my best self when raising my child, but I didn't understand why.

As I continued to art journal about it, it became crystal clear that I enjoyed the child-rearing journey so much because I was so intentional about it. I mean, the stakes are definitely high when you're raising another human, another soul. But the high stakes were what made the journey enjoyable; the purpose—the "why"—was so clearly defined.

So, I could finally grasp my truth from "enjoy the journey." Now when I see it on a mug at Target, I can understand it at the heart level, the spiritual level, where to truly "enjoy the journey," we need to be intentional about it and its purpose in our lives.

I couldn't have gained that insight without my art journal.

FIFTEEN

YOUR JOURNEY TO SELF-DISCOVERY AND YOUR ART JOURNAL

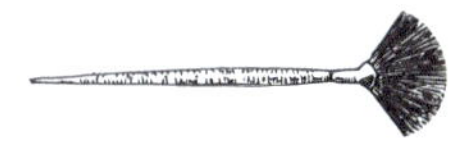

SINCE WE'RE ON THE TOPIC OF CLICHÉ QUOTES, THERE'S ANOTHER ONE that you're probably familiar with: "Life is a journey." My question to myself back then and now to you is this: Is it really life that's the journey, or is it the self-discovery that happens throughout our lives? Personally, I consider self-discovery to be a way of travel—a trip through time, our minds, our hearts, and our spirits. In fact, self-discovery is a pilgrimage of sorts, where we diverge from the pressures of society and silence the opinions of our family and friends to learn what we really feel about ourselves and our priorities.

My art journal is my guide on my ongoing journey to self-discovery. I use it as a telescope to look forward in times of transition and a microscope to examine inward in times of intense emotion.

I also use it as a journey map to look back on my life to identify patterns and themes that keep recurring in my present tense. After all, they say that hindsight is 20-20, right? Over time, an art journal becomes a visual narrative of our personal journey.

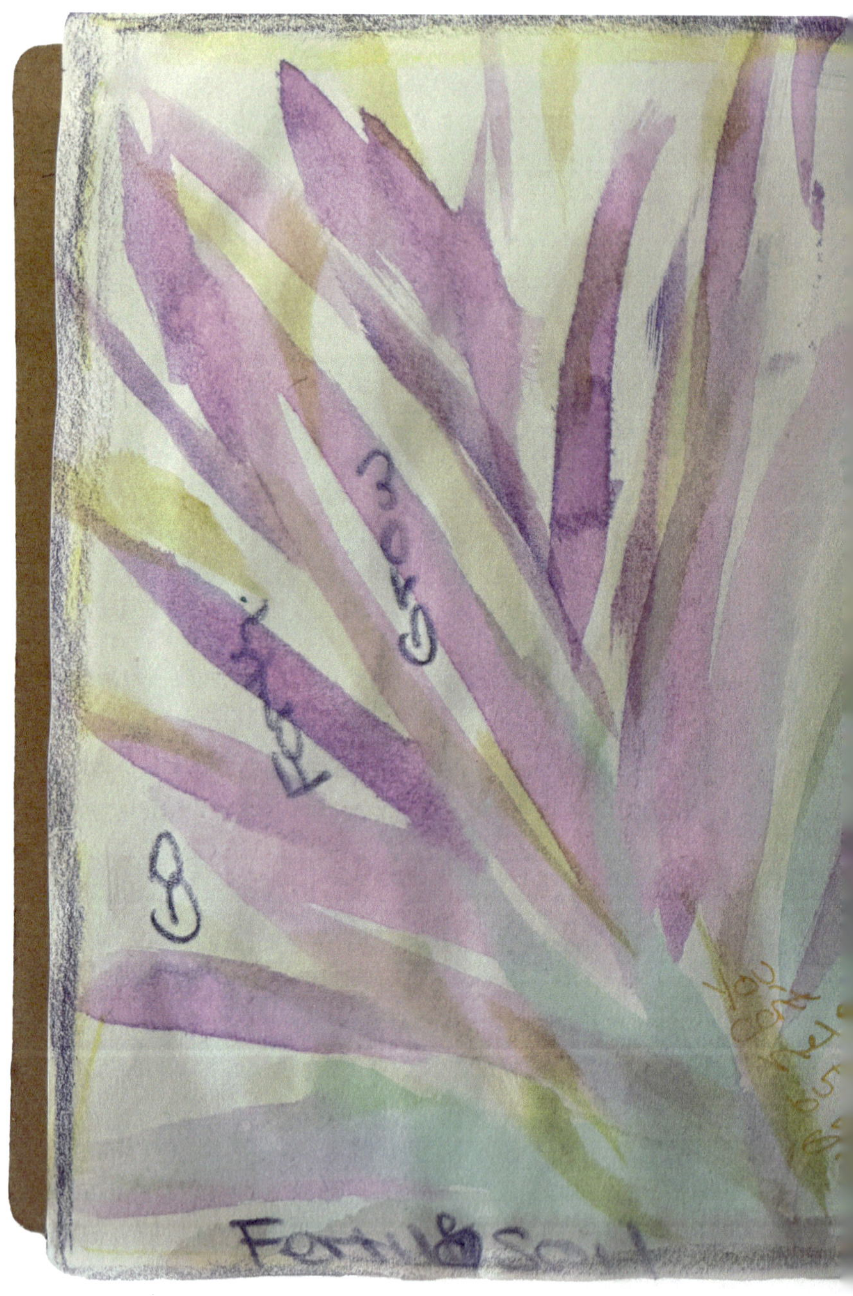

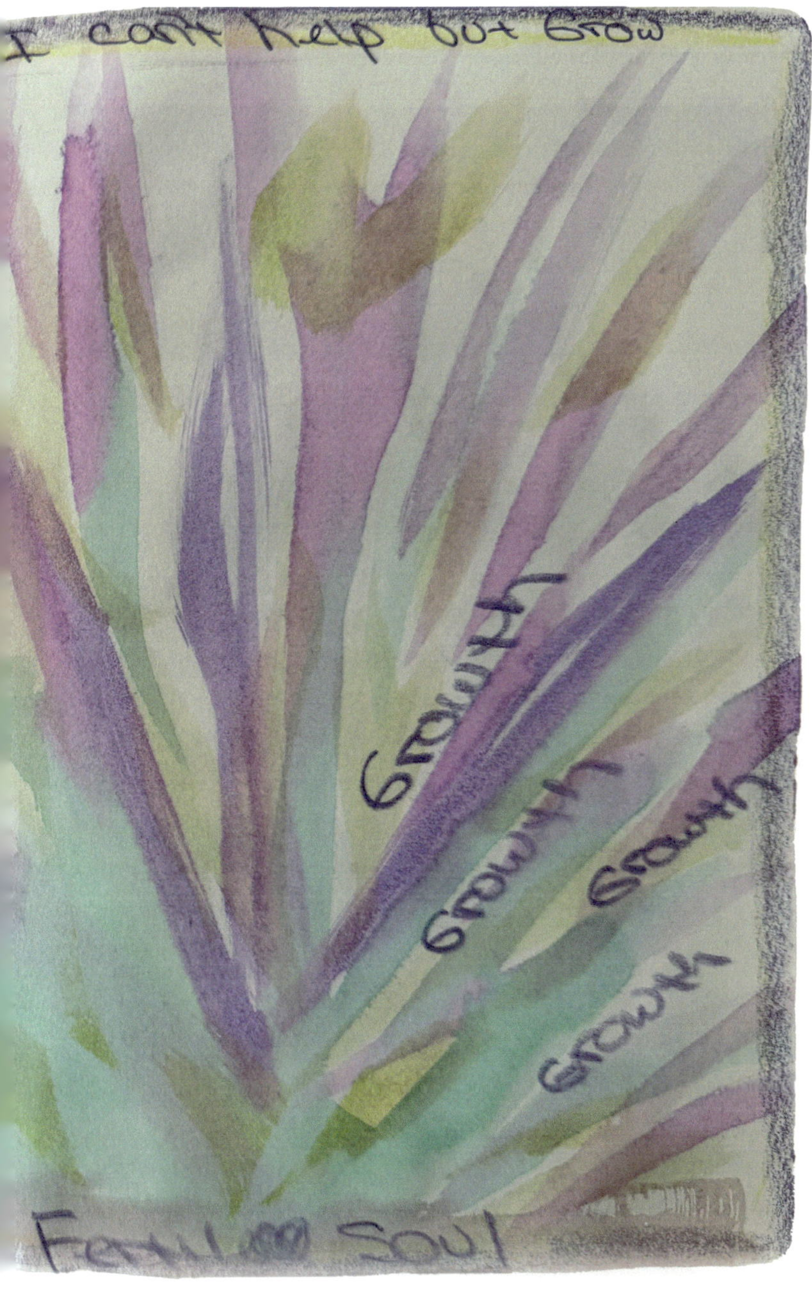

Your thoughts and ideas can translate into the physical movement of the brush, pen, or pencil, creating a unique pattern or image that captures the thought. In this example, growth.

Looking back at previous entries can reveal patterns, progress, and changes in perspective, aiding in self-reflection, growth, and ultimately, self-discovery.

"The universe is full of magic things patiently waiting for our senses to become sharper."
—EDEN PHILLPOTTS

Leo Tolstoy is said to have said, "The two most powerful warriors are patience and time." The quote makes me think of how the pages of my art journal create the space that only patience and time can. I can create shapes and colors on a page in the heat of the moment. Then, days, weeks, or even years later, I can look back at the page as a snapshot in time. It's as if my art journal is a time-traveling journal documenting my thoughts and emotions over time. So, the colors and shapes on the page create a freeze frame, or snapshot, of what I was feeling in the moment, and then later, on a day when I'm feeling anxious, fearful, or agitated, I can revisit those past pages, and the time and patience of the journal pieces give me perspective. I can view the pages in the context of what happened before, during, and after I created them. The colors, media, and arrangement of each page capture the event and its impact on me. Armed with that perspective, I have the ability to say, "Oh, this icky feeling is part of a pattern, or it's a common theme triggered by certain situations." Then I can explore that long-held pattern and determine if I need to change anything about myself or how I handle certain events.

For example, I can say to myself that [insert image] was created during a time when I was feeling [insert feeling]. At the time, it was hard to see the big picture because I was stuck in [insert reaction] at the moment. But later, when I looked back at that page, I thought, "Oh yeah, I remember that. Turns out it wasn't the end of the world;

I was just reacting to [this event] with [that emotion]." And, *voilà*, pattern detected!

I encourage you to look back on your journal pages to see if you can identify patterns and trends. You might be seriously surprised to find that the simple combinations of colors and shapes hold multitudes of wisdom.

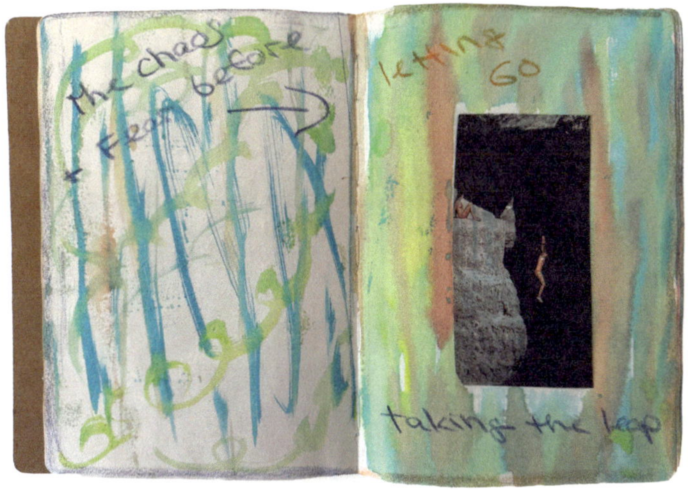

More cliffs, more jumping.

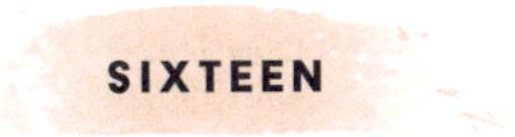

SIXTEEN

INTEGRATE MIND AND BODY

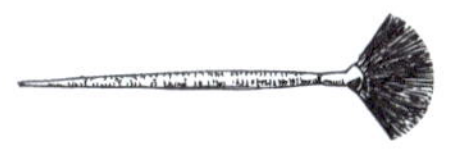

"Wherever we are, we can take a deep breath, feel our body, open our senses and step outside the endless stories of the mind."

—JACK KORNFIELD

BECAUSE MY ART JOURNALING SERVES AS A BRIDGE BETWEEN MY conscious and subconscious mind—my right brain and left brain—looking at the pages in retrospect helps me to integrate my mind and body, too. Looking back at my journal, I can tie trends in my physical state of being to specific triggers. It's all documented in the pages of my journal. It's all about pattern recognition.

For example, I started to have lower back pain in 2021. In fact, the pains started in earnest on the very first day of 2021. Because the pain was in my lower back, I assumed it was related to my pandemic-induced New Year's resolution to do push-ups every day.

The back pains led to stomach pains, which then led to chest pains. They really freaked me out. There were some nights that my anxiety was so bad that I wondered if I would wake up in the morn-

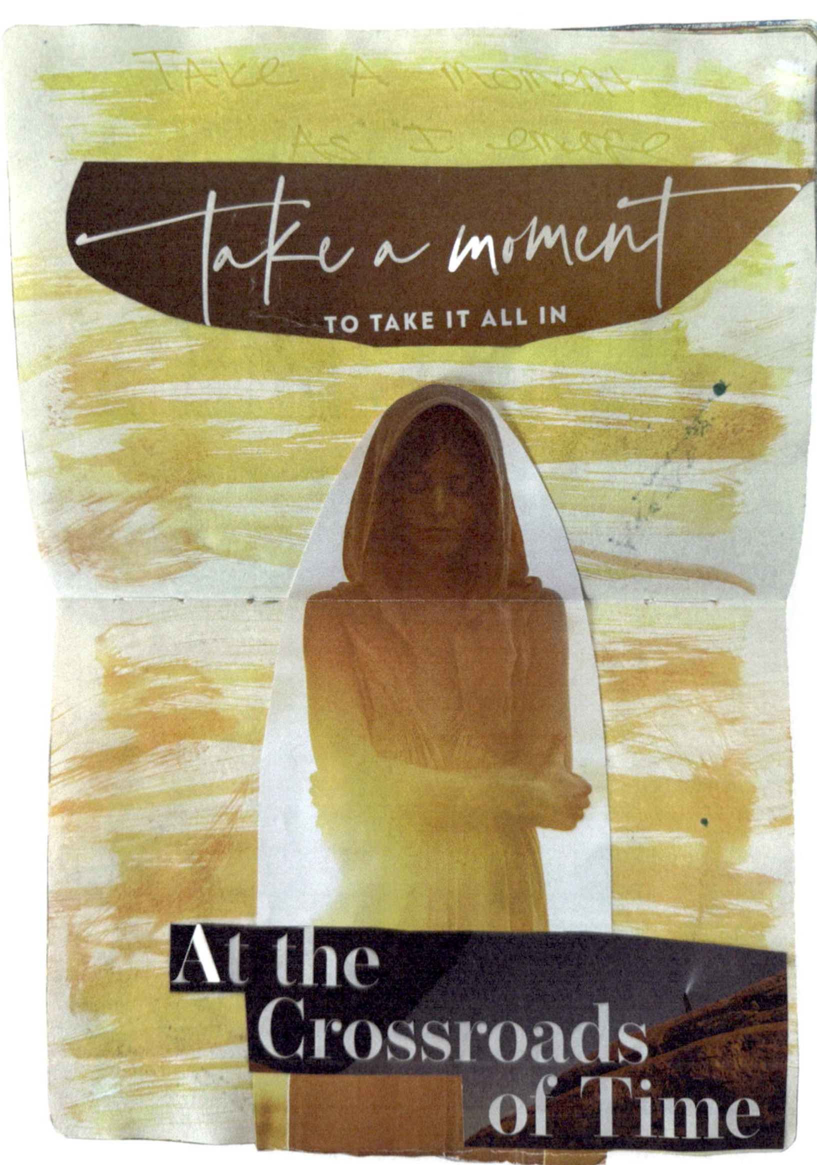

I had saved this image for months. On this particular day, with the release and peace I felt, I knew it was time to put her in my journal.

ing. I even asked myself, am I dying? The answer was always not now, not today.

Okay…but what, then?

I would chase the pains with internet searches, which it turns out, is the absolutely worst thing to do when having medical problems. I would doom-scroll through pages and pages of terrifying potentialities delivered by the dismal search results.

I saw lots of doctors and got lots of tests during that time. Thankfully, all showed that I was healthy. But there is something so incredibly unhelpful about a normal test, right?

The question remained: What were these pains?

Well, after a while, it was clear that the doctors were stumped and had reached a dead end. Discouraged and still anxious, I turned to my art journal out of habit. As I colored and made collages, answers began to take shape.

As I said, the pandemic was a gut-wrenching time, and according to my art journal, the impact of it was literally wrenching my body, creating these mysterious but very real pains. In that I'm an empath, which I've always known, the situation was like a double dose of high-fructose sugar. Empaths, by nature, take a lot in and hold a lot of emotion for others. I am both sympathetic and empathic, and it became clear through my pages that I was taking on too much that wasn't mine. My husband has heart problems, and I would feel his problems; the pandemic world felt topsy-turvy, so I was topsy-turvy. Add all that uneasiness to the fact that I had spent the last two years constantly second-guessing my sensory abilities (Can I taste this? Can I smell that?) in order to catch the cardinal signs of the COVID-19 virus. It was like trying to drink from a fire hose. My nervous system was on overdrive, and I was feeling everything. It all was passing through my body.

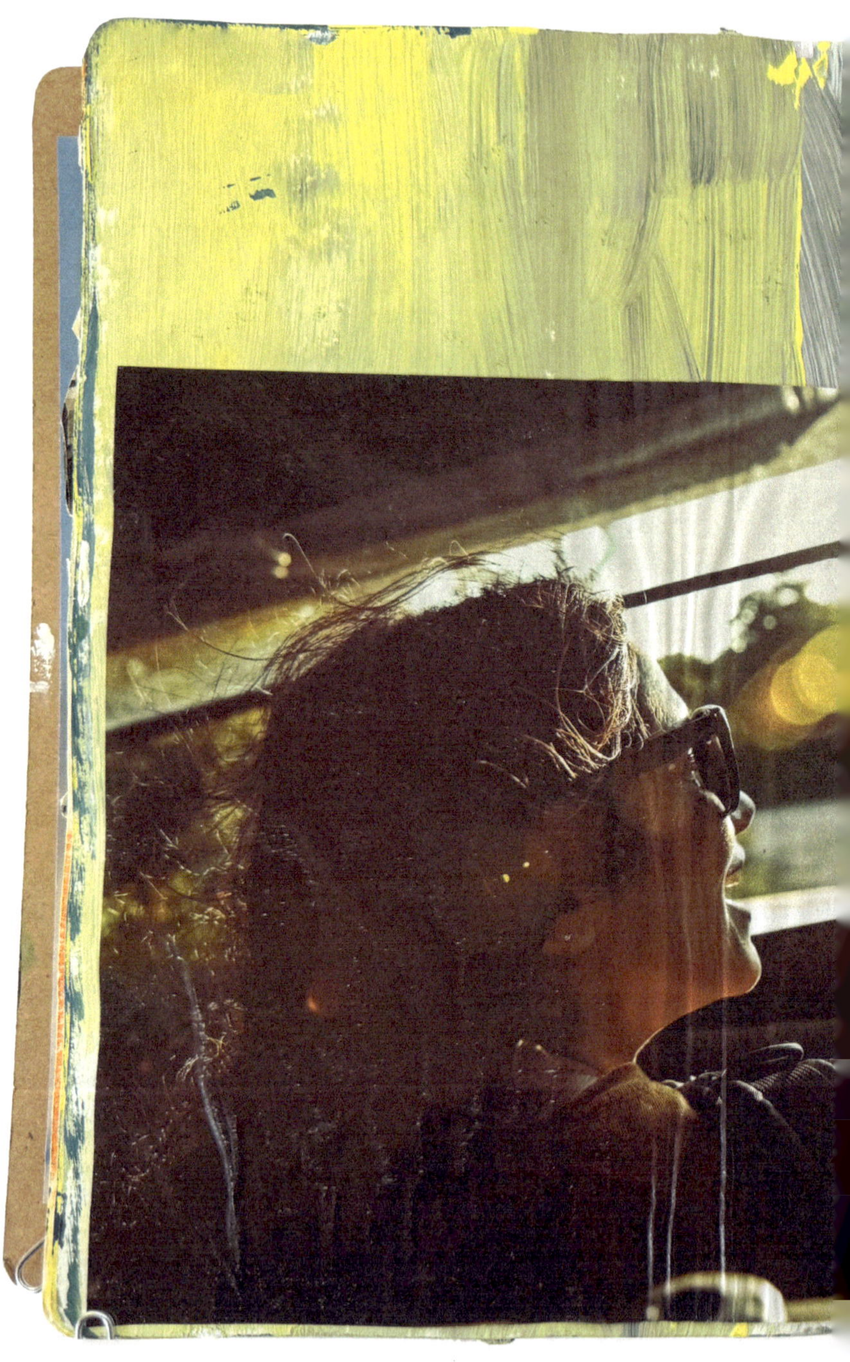

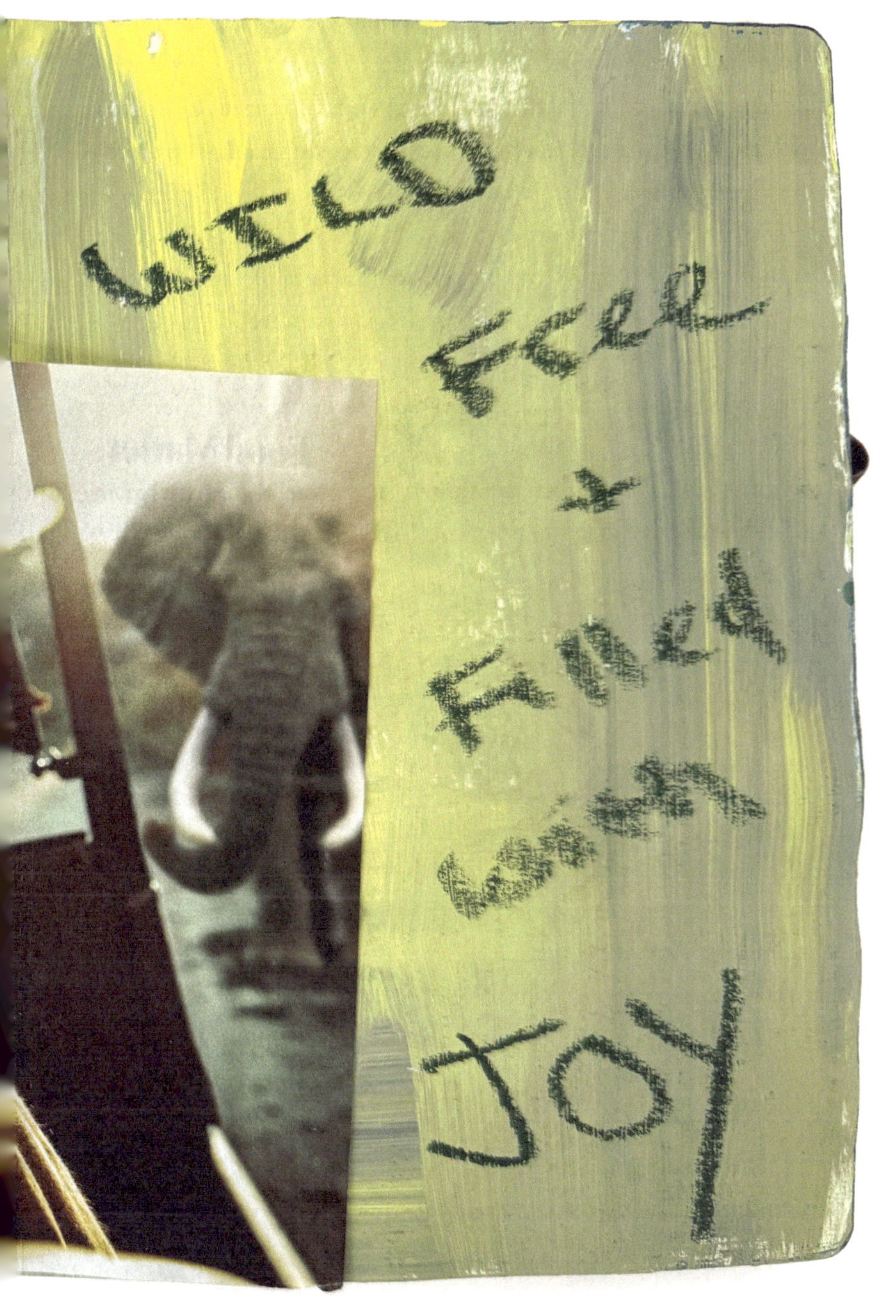

Thanks to my inner artist, "Wild, Free, and Filled with Joy" became my mantra during this period.

The art journal helped me to make that connection, easing my mind. The thorough workup from my doctors and seeing previously hidden patterns of stress and anxiety in my art journal ultimately provided me with a more complete understanding of how my body was talking to me.

Now when I listen to my body, I can get out of my worry loop and into creating pages in my journal that capture the conflict, chaos, and more and more often unbounded joy I am feeling.

I say give art journaling at a try and let that four-year-old artist out to color and draw. Through it, I'm sure you will not only have some playtime but also learn so much about your body, mind, and spirit. You also can let me know if it's made a difference in your life at susan@susan-hensley.com. I'd love to hear such stories from my readers.

"The mind can go in a thousand directions, but on this beautiful path, I walk in peace. With each step, a gentle wind blows. With each step, a flower blooms."

—THICH NHAT HANH

By now you're ready to create on your own, but let's take a moment together and just breathe deeply, feeling your body. Slowly scan through your body as you breathe, starting at your head and gently, patiently working down to your toes.

What do you feel? You can just observe the sensation whatever it may be—tight, clenching, tingly—we all are unique, so just observe your experience. After you have observed your body, pull out your journal and capture what you felt, what you heard your inner voice say, and any areas that want your attention. Create playfully without judgment.

ACKNOWLEDGMENTS

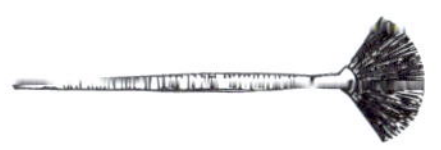

I AM DEEPLY GRATEFUL TO EVERYONE WHO CONTRIBUTED TO THE creation of *Art for Your Sanity* and supported me along the way.

First and foremost, I want to express my heartfelt appreciation to my husband, Bob, for his unwavering support and encouragement throughout this journey. Your love and belief in me have been my greatest motivation and without which this book would not have come to fruition. To my parents, for their inspiration. My mom as an author showing me what is possible, and to my dad for his love of art and design. And of course, to my son, Brent, for motivating me to be the best version of myself since the day he was born.

I extend my gratitude to my close circle of friends. Kristi, who has consistently showed me the way through her humor, love, and patience, and Amy and Margret for their valuable insights and encouragement as I navigated this process. To Adele, whose passion for art and willingness to share her hobby introduced me to making an art journal in the first place. To my book club for the richness you bring to life and support we give one another.

A special thank you to the teams at MEA and Canyon Ranch for the work they do helping people explore their purpose and passions, and to Martha Beck whose in person and online courses kept me taking one small step at a time.

I also want to acknowledge the support of the entire team at

Book Launchers, especially Erica and Kate, who worked tirelessly to bring this book to life. Your professionalism and dedication have been instrumental in shaping its final form.

Lastly, to the readers who embarked on this journey with me, thank you for your trust and willingness to explore the power of art journaling as a tool for personal growth and resilience.

With deepest gratitude,

Susan

APPENDIX

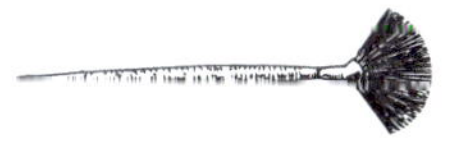

Ashdown, Brien K., Jamie S. Bodenlos, Kelsey Marie Arroyo, Melanie Patterson, Elena Parkins, and Sarah Burstein. "How Does Coloring Influence Mood, Stress, and Mindfulness?" *Journal of Integrated Social Sciences* 8, no. 1 (2018): 1–21, https://www.jiss.org/documents/volume_8/JISS%202018%208(1)%20 1-21%20Coloring%20and%20Mindfulness.pdf.

Martha Beck (@themarthabeck). "Everything is changing. Everything feels strange. No one knows what's coming next. In the midst of all this, what should you do now?" Instagram caption, January 3, 2024. https://www.instagram.com/themarthabeck/p/C1p3McHrQtu/.

Brown, Brené. *Atlas of the Heart: Mapping Meaningful Connection and the Language of Human Experience.* New York: Random House, 2021.

Des Marais, Saya. "The Importance of Play for Adults." Last modified November 10, 2022. https://psychcentral.com/blog/the-importance-of-play-for-adults.

Dixon, Travis. "What Is 'Enculturation?'" IB Psychology, June 20, 2017. https://www.themantic-education.com/ib-psych/2017/06/20/what-is-enculturation/.

Eaton, Judy, and Christine Tieber. "The Effects of Coloring on Anxiety, Mood, and Perseverance." *Art Therapy*, 35, no. 1 (2017): 42–46. https://doi.org/10.1080/07421656.2016.1277113.

Götz, Ignacio L. "On Defining Creativity." *The Journal of Aesthetics and Art Criticism* 39, no. 3 (1981): 297–301. https://doi.org/10.2307/430164.

Let's Talk: How to Improve Your Mental Health Through Duality." Trellis Society. Accessed February 3, 2024. https://www.growwithtrellis.ca/stories/mental-health-duality.

Magsamen, Susan, and Ivy Ross. *Your Brain on Art: How the Arts Transform Us*. New York: Penguin Random House. 2023.

Magnuson, Carl D., and Lynn A. Barnett. "The Playful Advantage: How Playfulness Enhances Coping with Stress." *Leisure Sciences*, 35, no. 2 (2013) 129–144. https://doi.org/10.1080/01490400.2013.761905.

"Study Reveals Global Creativity Gap." Adobe. April 23, 2010. https://news.adobe.com/news/news-details/2012/Study-Reveals-Global-Creativity-Gap/default.aspx.

Taylor, Jill Bolte. *Whole Brain Living: The Anatomy of Choice and the Four Characters That Drive Our Life*. New York: Penguin Random House. 2022.

Thiel, Ansgar, Hendrik K. Thedinga, Samantha L. Thomas, Harald Barkhoff, Katrin E. Giel, Olesia Schweizer, Syra Thiel, and Stephan Zipfel. "Have Adults Lost Their Sense of Play? An Observational Study of the Social Dynamics of Physical (In)activity in German and Hawaiian Leisure Settings." *BMC Public Health* 16, no. 689. https://doi.org/10.1186/s12889-016-3392-3.

van der Kolk, Bessel A. *The Body Keeps the Score: Brain, Mind, and Body in the Healing of Trauma*. New York: Viking Press (2014).

Vocabulary.com Dictionary, s.v. "duality." Accessed February 05, 2024. https://www.vocabulary.com/dictionary/duality.

Made in the USA
Columbia, SC
31 December 2024

50953408R00061